EVIDENCE-BASED TEACHING IN NURSING

A Foundation for Educators

SHARON CANNO

Regional Dean/

Center of Excellence i

Texas Tech Universit

School

Odes

CAROL BOSWELL,

Professor/C

Center of Excellence i

Texas Tech Universit

School

Ode:

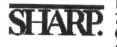
JONES
L E A

World Headquarters

Jones & Bartlett Learning
40 Tall Pine Drive
Sudbury, MA 01776
978-443-5000
info@jblearning.com
www.jblearning.com

Jones & Bartlett Learning
Canada
6339 Ormindale Way
Mississauga, Ontario L5V 1J2
Canada

Jones & Bartlett Learning
International
Barb House, Barb Mews
London W6 7PA
United Kingdom

Jones & Bartlett Learning books and products are available through most bookstores and online booksellers. To contact Jones & Bartlett Learning directly, call 800-832-0034, fax 978-443-8000, or visit our website, www.jblearning.com.

Substantial discounts on bulk quantities of Jones & Bartlett Learning publications are available to corporations, professional associations, and other qualified organizations. For details and specific discount information, contact the special sales department at Jones & Bartlett Learning via the above contact information or send an email to specialsales@jblearning.com.

The authors, editor, and publisher have made every effort to provide accurate information. However, they are not responsible for errors, omissions, or for any outcomes related to the use of the contents of this book and take no responsibility for the use of the products and procedures described. Treatments and side effects described in this book may not be applicable to all people; likewise, some people may require a dose or experience a side effect that is not described herein. Drugs and medical devices are discussed that may have limited availability controlled by the Food and Drug Administration (FDA) for use only in a research study or clinical trial. Research, clinical practice, and government regulations often change the accepted standard in this field. When consideration is being given to use of any drug in the clinical setting, the health care provider or reader is responsible for determining FDA status of the drug, reading the package insert, and reviewing prescribing information for the most up-to-date recommendations on dose, precautions, and contraindications, and determining the appropriate usage for the product. This is especially important in the case of drugs that are new or seldom used.

Production Credits
Publisher: Kevin Sullivan
Acquisitions Editor: Amy Sibley
Associate Editor: Patricia Donnelly
Editorial Assistant: Rachel Shuster
Production Manager: Carolyn F. Rogers
Marketing Manager: Meagan Norlund
Associate Marketing Manager: Katie Hennessy
V.P., Manufacturing and Inventory Control: Therese Connell
Composition: Shepherd, Inc.
Cover Design: Scott Moden
Cover Image: © Marilyn Volan/ShutterStock, Inc.
Printing and Binding: Malloy, Inc.
Cover Printing: Malloy, Inc.

Library of Congress Cataloging-in-Publication Data
Cannon, Sharon, 1940-
    Evidence-based teaching in nursing : a foundation for educators / Sharon
Cannon, Carol Boswell.
        p. ; cm.
    Includes bibliographical references and index.
    ISBN 978-0-7637-8575-8 (pbk.)
    1. Nursing—Study and teaching. 2. Teaching—Methodology.
3. Evidence-based nursing. I. Boswell, Carol. II. Title.
    [DNLM: 1. Teaching—Methodology. 2. Education, Nursing—methods.
3. Evidence-Based Nursing—methods. WY 105]
    RT73.C29 2011
    610.73076—dc22
                                    2010037479
6048
Printed in the United States of America
15 14 13 12 11   10 9 8 7 6 5 4 3 2

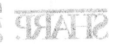

Contents

Preface

Evidence-based practice came upon the healthcare scene over 30 years ago. Although it is only within the last 10 to 15 years that evidence-based practice has gained in respect and importance, it has now reached a point of being expected for each and every health skill utilized. Members of the health team and public consumers understand the importance of utilizing healthcare skills and knowledge that are supported by strong evidence. Nursing schools have readily embraced the idea that all components of the program of study must reflect the value and use of evidence-based practice for the novice and expert nurse. Since indeed the idea is that all aspects of healthcare provision must reflect evidence-based practice, then of necessity, nursing education should embrace the same level of expertise: evidence-based teaching.

This textbook assimilates the ideas found within evidence-based practice as it endeavors to confront the initiative of evidence-based teaching. Education is paramount for the development of qualified, competent healthcare providers. The notion that education would not rise to the challenge of confirming the delivery of educational material through the use of evidence-supported principles is unthinkable. The educational field has accepted the idea that everyone "teaches as they were taught." We must move beyond this idea to utilizing teaching techniques and methodologies which are grounded in evidence.

Technological advancements, knowledgeable consumers of education, and well-informed clients of health care demand that nursing education keep pace and address our ever-changing world.

Each chapter in this text looks at different aspects of the educational process in light of the evidence. The initial five chapters develop a foundation on which to launch evidence-based teaching. Within these chapters, theories, legal aspects, role development, and definitions are provided for application to the educational environment. For each area, the evidence which is currently available is utilized. The next three chapters directly look at the nursing educational settings found—classroom, online, and clinical. Within each of these chapters, the evidence for different delivery methodologies is provided. Chapters 9 and 10 move to rounding out the idea of nursing education by looking at program evaluation and competency/certification. The final chapter challenges each of us to move evidence-based teaching into the next century. This chapter provides the challenge for every nursing faculty member to consider and embrace.

The contributors to this book are experts in the world of nursing education. It has been a privilege and honor to collaborate with each of them as we take this journey toward evidence-based teaching. It is our resolution and declaration that you will accept the challenge of evidence-based teaching and be invigorated by the potential for advancing the field of nursing education. Though evidence for the different aspects of the educational process is available, research evidence is insufficient. So, the other challenge which emerges from this textbook is the ultimatum that nursing educational research needs to be conducted to confirm or refute the different aspects of the educational process.

Sharon B. Cannon, EdD, RN, ANEF
Texas Tech University Health Sciences Center, School of Nursing
Odessa, Texas

Carol Boswell, EdD, RN, CNE, ANEF
Texas Tech University Health Sciences Center, School of Nursing
Odessa, Texas

Acknowledgments

As opportunities come available and challenges are identified, pathways are found that allow each of us to stretch and grow. We are provided the destiny to step out and look at our environment from different viewpoints. Following the energies put toward evidence-based practice aspects, the natural progression was to apply those same ideas and concepts to the field of nursing education. We would like to take this opportunity to communicate our appreciation to our extraordinary and visionary colleagues who took this trip with us to clarify and refine the idea of evidence-based teaching. In addition to our students who challenge us to be visionary, timely, and real, we express our heartfelt appreciation for the opportunity to begin a journey and to strive for excellence.

Dr. Sharon Cannon and Dr. Carol Boswell

When I started as a young nurse, I never in my wildest dreams imagined that I would or could be where I am today. My parents, Babe and Laurine Cannon, provided the motivation and support for me to continue my education and most of all gave me a love for learning. My brother and his wife, Gene and Cathie Cannon, have been and continue to be a source and comfort over the years and, without even being aware, continue to carry on my parents' legacy for education. In addition, my son, Ryan Ganey, and my daughter, Lynn Tischner, and her husband, Joe Tischner, always keep me looking to the future and are always there with encouragement and love. My beautiful grandchildren, Kelly Tischner, Andrew, Shelby, and Shannon Ganey are the bright stars that will shine for me in the years to come.

My professional life has been blessed by mentors who helped to guide me to seek opportunities that would challenge me and stretch my skills and abilities far beyond the goals I had established. Dr. Shirley Martin and Dr. Martha Welch may not have any idea of the impact they have had on my nursing career. Finally, one mentor, colleague, and friend—Dr. Carol Boswell—is a treasure. She keeps me on the "straight and narrow" and she is the sister of my dreams in so many ways. With all of that in mind, I wish for each of you to have the support, love, and encouragement that I have had bestowed upon me in my life. May you seek the evidence and let it take you to newer heights to fulfill your dreams.

Dr. Sharon Cannon

As a parent, the frustration of hearing the continuous question "WHY?" has resulted in my commitment to address the "why" query prior to it being asked whenever possible. We all desire to understand the rationale for why we are doing things. As an educator, the dedication to discerning and acknowledging the reasons and justifications has led me down this path to evidence-based teaching. So to my children (Michael Boswell, Casey Boswell, Jeremy Boswell, and Stephanie Boswell) and my grandchildren (Matthew Boswell, Kobe Boswell, Kayia Howard, and Caleb Boswell), keep challenging me to answer the questions of: why tasks are required, what is the reason for taking a path, and where do we go from here. To my husband (Marc E. Boswell) and my mother (Wanda Miller), thank you for your continuing support as I delve into new ventures and strive for different heights. To the nursing students who are engaged and excited about learning, my genuine indebtedness makes me do my homework to better serve you as you strive for excellence in nursing care and to further your education. Finally, my mentor and friend (Dr. Sharon Cannon) allows me ample opportunities to brainstorm about creative and futurist ideas. Our brainstorming sessions allow me to reach for the stars and seek new directions. Thank you for encouraging me to strive for the stars and hold fast to innovative thoughts. Without the encouragement and steadfastness of my family, friends, and students, I would not be able to brave the challenges of the educational and nursing communities while embracing the legitimacy of what is significant and essential within a person's being.

Dr. Carol Boswell

Contributors

Theresa M. "Terry" Valiga, EdD, RN, ANEF, FAAN
Director, Institute for Educational Excellence
Clinical Professor
School of Nursing
Duke University
Durham, NC

Linda Caputi, EdD, RN, CNE
Professor Emeritus
College of DuPage
Glen Ellyn, IL

Joyce M. Miller, DNP, RN, WNHP-BC
Assistant Professor
Anita Thigpen Perry School of Nursing
Texas Tech University Health Sciences Center
Odessa, TX

Patricia Allen, EN, EdD, CNE, ANEF
Professor and Director, Center for Innovation in Nursing Education
Texas Tech University Health Sciences Center
Lubbock, TX

Chapter 1

Overview of Evidence-Based Practice

Carol Boswell and Sharon Cannon

Chapter Objectives

At the conclusion of this chapter, the learner will be able to:

1. Discuss the differences between evidence-based practice and evidence-based teaching.
2. Identify the evolution of evidence-based practice within health care.
3. Explain key aspects of critical thinking.
4. State the specific steps involved in evidence-based teaching.
5. List the steps needed to conduct a literature review to find evidence related to a teaching/learning topic.

Key Terms

- ➤ Critical thinking
- ➤ Evidence-based practice
- ➤ Evidence-based teaching
- ➤ PSCOT format

Introduction

As nursing continues its migration toward professionalism and advancement of the profession, the idea of scholarship becomes increasingly important. The American Association of Colleges of Nursing (AACN) stated that "scholarship in nursing can be defined as those activities that systematically advance the teaching, research, and practice of nursing through rigorous inquiry that (1) is significant to the profession, (2) is creative, (3) can be documented, (4) can be replicated or elaborated, and (5) can be peer-reviewed through various methods" (1999, para. 5). With the confirmation of **evidence-based practice** (EBP) as a foundational aspect within nursing, the idea of methodically and analytically strengthening the fundamental principles while advancing scholarship to move evidence-based practice toward **evidence-based teaching** (EBT) is judicious and appropriate. According to Shultz (2009), "developing the science of nursing education is a journey that involves many individuals and many activities. It is a never-ending task that incorporates the continual asking of questions and the ongoing search for understanding" (p. 302). Careful steps and strategies for assimilating the multiplexity of the teaching/learning process require that each of us stay vigilant in asking the right questions. The other side of the coin requires that nursing faculty members stay committed to the lifelong pursuit of knowledge.

The healthcare community has embraced the idea and expectation for EBP. The different activities that are assumed within healthcare delivery are expected to be based upon the best evidence that is available. Can we expect anything less when we move into the area of teaching/learning? Wexler (n.d.) makes an interesting and true statement: "All the rhetoric about passionate teaching, and whether professors care about or value teaching, is meaningless if they are bad or ineffective teachers" (para 4). Moving away from the idea that anyone can teach and toward the concept that effective and productive teaching must be founded on sound, defensible strategies becomes the battle cry. No longer can academia accept mediocre teaching. Our battle cry must be "Effective Teaching results in Successful Learning." The nursing education community must ensure that the strategies and practices incorporated into the classroom and the learning environment are firmly founded on the best evidence as to what improves the acquisition of knowledge.

Boyer (1990) stated that "we believe the time has come to move beyond the tired old 'teaching versus research' debate and give the familiar and honorable term 'scholarship' a broader, more capacious meaning, one that brings legitimacy to the full scope of academic work" (p. 16). The handiwork of the scholar requires each of us to step back from only encouraging an individual's exploration and move toward networking, constructing connections between theory and practice, and communicating knowledge efficiently to students and others. The process of bringing each of the multiple threads together to form a beautiful tapestry of teaching and learning necessitates the scholar to organize and conceptualize the components based upon the best evidence available. It requires willingness to try new ideas and struggle with the process while keeping an eye on the goal of improving the educational process. Shultz (2009) summarizes the ideas in the statement: "Every faculty member can contribute to the development of the science of nursing education by searching for evidence to support the teaching strategies and evaluation methods to be used in their courses and talking with colleagues about gaps in our knowledge when such evidence is not found" (p. 302). Each and every one of us must accept the responsibility to strive for innovative avenues to engage the student and transfer the knowledge needed to result in competent healthcare providers.

Historical Perspectives

The nursing process has been at the foundation of nursing practice for well over three decades. The profession of nursing has begun to look beyond this foundation toward knowledge based upon a firm underpinning of evidence. Malloch and Porter-O'Grady (2006) termed this movement forward as *disciplined clinical inquiry* (DCI). Disciplined clinical inquiry provided nurses with alternatives that allowed learning and engagement with the knowledge available, as it applied to nontraditional settings. The concept of disciplined clinical inquiry evolved into the current term **critical thinking**. As the profession was challenged to base the provision of care on sound knowledge supported by evidence, the inspiration for EBP was born.

Evidence-based practice was first acknowledged in the 1970s. It was during this time period that different people from different areas realized that the practice of health care needed to be established on the facts, rather than just what had been done for years. Dr. Archie Cochrane, a British physician, has gained the distinction of being the pioneer and inspiration for the evidence-based medicine movement. As a result of his ground-breaking work in 1972, the Cochrane Center in Oxford, England, was established in 1992 and the Cochrane Collaboration was recognized in 1993. The premise for the Cochrane Collaboration is to advance healthcare decision making through the use of systematic reviews concerning the outcome of evidence from healthcare interventions. The Cochrane Collaboration and Center are international, not-for-profit, independent organizations that are committed to ensuring that state-of-the-art, accurate information concerning the outcomes of healthcare interventions is accessible by the global community.

Following in the footsteps provided by Dr. Cochrane, several nursing leaders transformed the principles to address the profession of nursing. Evidence-based nursing practice models are numerous. Each of the models was formulated to address a key aspect within the nursing practice. The Stetler model was one of the initial prototypes to be established. It was formulated in 1976 as a research utilization model. This version of EBP was initiated as a practitioner-oriented model with a concentration on critical thinking and individual use of the findings. Another well-known international collaboration within EBP and nursing is the Joanna Briggs Institute. This institute was established in 1996 for use by nurses, medical and allied health researchers, clinicians, academicians, and quality managers. The Joanna Briggs Institute is utilized in over 40 countries and on every continent. The centralized impetus for this institute is to establish the usefulness, suitability, meaningfulness, and practicability related to health routine, tradition, and healthcare delivery approaches. A third EBP model, developed in 1999, is the Rosswurn-Larrabee model. This model is based upon the use of theoretical and research literature. It is used to guide practitioners toward the effective utilization of EBP.

In the last 10 years, several nursing EBP models have been showcased. The Iowa Model was established to assist the clinician at the bedside in the acute care setting to utilize a practical EBP organizational model. Within this model, triggers are used to assist the bedside nurse to take the steps to carefully consider the clinical decision-making process as he or she delivers EBP care. The Advancing Research and Clinical Practice Through Close Collaboration (ARCC) model was established to help advance practice nurses to implement EBP successfully. With the ARCC model, the idea of establishing a network of clinicians who are willing to disseminate best evidence and to function as champions for EBP is the foundational support for this model. Another EBP model to consider is called the ACESTAR model. This model originates from the idea of knowledge transformation. It attempts to comprehend the sequences, essence, and characteristics of knowledge. These models are a few of the many EBP models that can be found and used in the clinical provision of health care; furthermore, new models are being developed to address key aspects and applications of EBP.

Though these models are developing and escalating, evidence-based teaching (EBT) models are not found. The concepts and ideas considered in relationship to EBT are noted within the literature but actual models of how to do EBT are not found. It appears that the accepted attitude leans toward the idea that the models for EBP are enough. With the idea that teaching and learning strategies should be established based on valid and reliable evidence, the application of evidence-based principles directly related to teaching becomes increasingly important. According to Emerson and Records (2008), "the practice of nursing education is that which we do, including teaching didactic and clinical courses, advising students, and designing curricula, as well as our programs of study and the environments in which they are conducted" (p. 359). The teaching/learning environment includes the entire community that comes into play within the teaching/learning experience. The process of EBT must address all of the facets that impact the educational process (**Figure 1-1**). Danielson

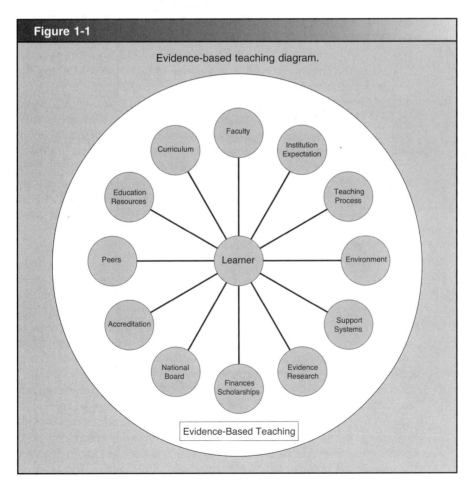

Figure 1-1

Evidence-based teaching diagram.

(2008) presents an important idea that "meaningful conversations about teaching and valid evaluation of teaching must be grounded in a clear definition of practice—a framework for teaching" (para 1). As we evolve the idea of EBT, a dialogue pertaining to the multifaceted aspects integrated into the acquisition of knowledge within the educational community will be initiated and followed.

Steps of EBP with Application to EBT

Evidence-based practice has been growing in popularity and functionality for many years. As we begin to move this concept into the area of Evidence-Based Teaching (EBT), several aspects need to be carefully considered. The definitions of EBP are numerous, so when you then consider EBT, even more problems arise. Is the definition of EBT different from that of EBP? If so, then how? Is finding a unique definition for EBT just splitting hairs? How is EBT different from EBP? In addition to the definition, the process of doing EBT also has unique characteristics that move it beyond the idea of EBP. Whereas EBP works within the clinical realm, EBT resides within a multiplicity of settings, which can include the clinical realm. Teaching is part of the work within the clinical space domain, but it does not take place only within that sphere. Teaching can and does take many different directions. According to Emerson and Records (2008), "the ultimate imperative facing nursing today is the creation of a culture that values the practice of nursing education and expands evidence-based education through the design, testing, and refinement of education strategies from nursing and other disciplines" (p. 359). The concepts and practices embodied within EBP must be applied to the system of nursing education. The steps and definitions applied to the management of EBP must be tailored to meet the expectations and actions embodied within the delivery of nursing education.

As a person begins to look deeply into the topic of EBP, multiple definitions can be found. These definitions somewhat address the same areas of concern but each has a unique focus. According to Boswell and Cannon (2011), the constant characteristics that are found within the multiple definitions relate to the decision-making scheme, clinical application, provider expertise, and client contribution. **Table 1-1** lists several definitions of EBP along with their related characteristics to provide an overview of the challenge in trying to reach a common definition. Each of the nursing EBP models seems to have a focal point, such as academia advanced nursing practice, bedside nursing care, and so forth. The definition used for the model is then aimed at addressing the aspects prevailing within that practice arena. Since there is not a common definition for EBP, the likelihood that a universal definition for EBT exists is next to impossible. Evidence-based teaching is just beginning to gain acceptance and support. Prior to this time period, the focus has been, and continues to be, aimed at ensuring that healthcare providers begin to understand and embrace the concepts of EBP. As different groups become increasingly comfortable with the EBP foundation, attempts to understand distinctive aspects such as teaching can be explored.

Several definitions for the scholarship of teaching are available for consideration as a definition for EBT is contemplated. According to the AACN (1999), "the scholarship of teaching is conducted through application of knowledge of the discipline or specialty area in the teaching-learning process, the development of innovative teaching and evaluation methods, program development, learning

Table 1-1

Evidence-Based Practice Definitions		
Source	Definition	Characteristics Noted
Melnyk & Fineout-Overholt, 2005	A process that permits healthcare providers to achieve the highest standard of care when managing the intricate needs of their patients and families.	Quality of care Multifaceted
Rutledge & Grant, 2002	Treatment that assimilates the top scientific data with clinical proficiency, knowledge of pathophysiology, knowledge of psychosocial concerns, and the decision-making processes of the clients.	Decision making Clinical focus Evidence Expertise Pathophysiology Psychosocial
Porter-O'Grady, 2006	The assimilation of the paramount research to evidence with clinical proficiency and with client requests.	Clinical focus Evidence Expertise Client involvement
Magee, 2005	The meticulous, unambiguous, and prudent utilization of existing preeminent evidence in formulating decisions about the treatment of a particular patient.	Decision making Evidence Client involvement
Pravikoff, Tanner, & Pierce, 2005	A methodical tactic of problem solving for healthcare providers exemplified by the employing of top data presently existing for clinical decision making to facilitate reliable and preeminent care to patients.	Decision making Clinical focus Evidence Client involvement
Boswell & Cannon, 2010	A method of employing established evidence (research and quality improvement), decision making, and nursing proficiency to regulate the provision of holistic client care.	Decision making Clinical focus Evidence Client involvement

outcome evaluations, and professional role modeling" (para 12). Each of these areas is viewed as an important theme that must be conscientiously considered as we endeavor to address teaching as a distinctive coordination of key hallmarks of excellence. The National League for Nursing (NLN) has not communicated a definition for EBT but has developed an Excellence in Nursing Education Model that depicts the different aspects central to the delivery of effective nursing education. The NLN took on the challenge of determining hallmarks of education and establishing academia as a unique discipline within the profession of nursing. This model can be viewed at www.nln.org/excellence/model/index.htm. The model covers the areas of student-centered, interactive, innovative programs and curricula; recognition of expertise; clear program standards and hallmarks that raise expectations; well-prepared faculty; qualified students; well-prepared educational administrators; evidence-based program and teaching/evaluation methods; and adequate, quality resources. For each area, the model further delineates multiple aspects to provide insight as to the different foci and facets that reflect the content within those areas.

Definitions for EBT are few in number. Emerson and Records (2008) define EBT practice in nursing as "the validation, generation, application, and perpetuation of those methods that facilitate the preparation of skilled and thoughtful nurses who function in a constantly evolving, global health care environment" (p. 361). It is interesting that within this definition the global aspect of health care is incorporated. Emerson and Records (2008) consider the integration of the responsibility of teaching with the scrutinization within teaching that embraces all of the roles and competencies from administrator to advisor to faculty. This definition reflects the idea that all aspects within the practice and management of the educational environment and process must be embedded in EBT.

Appling, Naumann, and Berk (2001) set forth the requirements subsumed within EBT as "the comprehensive measurement and evaluation of faculty teaching activities, with tools that capture multiple sources of evidence key to the accurate and complete measurement of teaching outcome" (p. 247). Within this definition, the focus of the process appears to be on the faculty and the classroom environment. Other aspects inherent in the academic environment and teaching routine are not evident in this definition. The evidence is intended for confronting the challenges faced within the classroom and learning ecosystem.

As each of these definitions for EBP and EBT is carefully considered and conceptualized, a working definition to be used within this text can be developed. For this text, EBT is a dynamic, holistic system using educational principles validated by evidence to support, maintain, and promote a new level of knowledge for a learner in a variety of settings. The process is viewed within a systems approach, and a "system is viewed as a group of interrelated, interacting, and/or interdependent constituents forming a complex whole" (*Webster's II New College Dictionary*, 1995, p. 1119). Each of the many different components within the EBT diagram (Figure 1-1) supports, interacts, and challenges the other components within the model. The learner is viewed as the center of the process within EBT. Each and every educational session and resource is intended to ensure that the learner is effectively placed in a position to gain the utmost knowledge from the educational environment. Though the individual learner is the center of the process, that center can also be represented by a cohort of learners.

The items within the diagram that network with and have effects on the learner during the educational process are faculty, institution expectations, teaching process, environment, support systems, evidence research, finances/scholarship, national board, accreditation, peers, education resources, and curriculum. When considering each of these items, faculty, curriculum, and peers are familiar aspects within the educational community. Institutional expectations can be viewed as the mission, philosophy, goals, and/or objectives established by the university or school. The aspects subsumed within the teaching processes are those strategies utilized within the educational process to deliver information. Another facet which affects the learner is the environment. The learning environment is a key feature which sets the stage for learning to occur. When the learning environment is stressful, disorganized, or threatening, the learner's ability to assimilate the information is compromised and impeded. Support systems are identified as another feature influencing the learner. Within this diagram, the support systems can include family, consulting services, health services, and other resources provided by the institution, community, or family for the students. On the other side of the diagram, the education resources are those measures such as tutoring services, testing departments, computer services, and so forth that are provided to aid in the delivery of instruction and the facilitation of the instructional process. An additional aspect which should impact the learner is the evidence supported by educational research. Each of these aspects should be founded on supporting evidence related to the feature. One more facet which has a large impact on the learner is the financial cost of acquiring an education. Within this aspect, the idea of scholarships, loans, and grants can play a part, as these different financial resources are used to support the learner's educational experience. The final two aspects are similar but occur at different levels. Accreditation concerns are frequently at the federal level and may be impacted by multiple agencies. National and state boards impact the learning process for several disciplines, nursing being just one.

Though each of these aspects has varying effects on the educational experience, each is viewed as important. Some of the aspects are more readily encountered by the learner, such as the faculty, teaching process, finances, peers, educational resources, and curriculum. Other aspects within the groups are of critical importance but may remain more in the background rather than being readily encountered during the day-to-day practice of the educational process. The holistic educational approach must address all of the aspects that impact the learner, such as peer support, curriculum, accreditation rules, and so forth. This approach is marked by continuous opportunities to evolve through the discovery and application of innovative evidence related to the teaching/learning process. The application of EBT to nursing is a multifaceted process that incorporates key components related to effective methodologies and roles to meet the needs of an ever-changing healthcare environment.

As a definition for EBT is resolved, the process then moves to the activities that are paramount to the successful management of the endeavor. **Figure 1-2** presents a visual depiction of the sequence embedded in the evolution of the process. The posing of the question is the crucial initial step for the initiation of an investigation into the evidence surrounding the educational process. The wording of the question must be clear and concise. By taking care to ensure that the question is effectively developed, the management of the literature review becomes increasingly more attainable. A well-developed question provides the key words and concepts imperative for identifying and narrowing the selection of the articles. By successfully ascertaining the articles through the literature search driven by the question, the evidence can be discovered which supports the teaching environment. The reviewing of these articles allows for the determination of EBT strategies. Many aspects—such as student values/preferences, student characteristics, academic boundaries, systematic evaluations, and financial/resource boundaries—come to bear on the teaching strategies. Within the synthesis of the evidence, each of these aspects along with other aspects must be carefully and systematically considered as the analysis of the evidence is completed.

Within the process of EBP, questions are presented in the PICOT format (**Table 1-2**). The PICOT format structures the question by looking at:

P = Population
I = Intervention(s)
C = Comparison(s)
O = Outcome(s)
T = Time

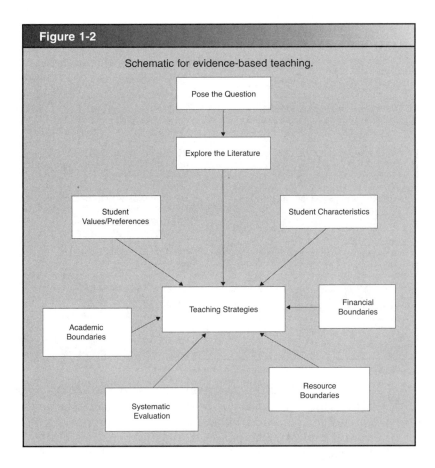

Figure 1-2

Schematic for evidence-based teaching.

By carefully examining each of these aspects, clarity and precision within the question are substantiated. Emerson and Records (2008) suggested the use of the STCO format for EBT questions. The STCO format includes:

S = Student
T = Teaching technique
C = Comparison
O = Outcome

Although this format provides focus to the educational aspects, it limits the population to students only. The educational process is much more than just the students. Many aspects within the educational process need to be founded upon evidence. Modifying the PICOT format to embrace the educational community results in increased continuity within the process of confirming evidence to

---

Table 1-2

Comparison of Evidence-Based Practice and Evidence-Based Teaching

Evidence-Based Practice	Evidence-Based Teaching
Ask the clinical question using the PICOT format: P (population), I (intervention), C (comparison), O (outcome), T (time)	Pose the education question using the PSCOT format: P (population), S (strategy), C (comparison), O (outcome), T (time)
Explore the evidence available to determine the best practice using a critical appraisal approach	Explore the evidence available to determine the best practice using a critical appraisal approach
Consider individual clinical expertise and client preferences/values as interventions are deliberated	Integrate teaching expertise with the students' characteristics, preferences, and values in the teaching/learning environment as solutions and ideas are formulated
Instigate clinical changes as needed within the parameters of the resources and stakeholders	Initiate educational modifications as needed within the academic, financial, and resource boundaries
Appraise the change in regard to patient satisfaction, financial considerations, institutional considerations, and professional considerations	Consider the changes based on key performance criteria identified with the systematic evaluation for the academic setting

Source: Adapted from Emerson, R. J., & Records, K. (2008). Today's challenge, tomorrow's excellence: The practice of evidence-based education. *Journal of Nursing Education, 47*(8), 359–370.

---

support best practices. As a result, the use of the **PSCOT format** can address the educational process. The "P" continues to be for the population. The population within the educational process can be directed toward students, administrators, faculty, alumni, candidates, preceptors, coaches, and many other groups of individuals who are involved in the educational process. The population can be either the individual or the cohort. Care needs to be given to understanding that within the academic arena, the student body or cohort may be viewed as the population instead of the individual student. As the population is designated, care must be given to narrowing the focus of the designation to allow for a clearer identification of the associates to be investigated. The "S" represents the educational strategy. Educational strategies are any aspect within the educational environment that comes into play for advancing the success of the learning process. Any intervention (strategy) that can affect the population must be carefully investigated to ensure that the overriding evidence is used to manage the learning environment for the betterment of the educational process. The "C" within the format mirrors the "C" within the EBP format. The incorporation of a comparison of educational strategies provides an evaluation of the different avenues for advancing the learning environment. Vigilantly looking at the different strategies within the context of the specific EBT question allows for determination of any divergence between the strategies. The "O" within the format also parallels the inclusion of outcome as used in the EBP format. As the EBT and EBP questions are posed, the identification of the expected outcomes allows the individual to clarify what is believed about the populations and the strategies being considered. The final aspect, the "T," within the question is the incorporation of the time period when applicable. Each and every question does not require the inclusion of the comparison nor a time setting, but it is helpful to clarify the question when used.

Let's look at some examples of PSCOT questions to see how the different aspects come into play in an EBT setting.

Example 1:
P = first semester students
S = use of care maps
C = use of care plans
O = improved pathology comprehension
T = (none used)

By looking at these different aspects, the question can be stated as: Do first-semester students who use care maps instead of care plans demonstrate an improved knowledge of the pathological aspect? Another example for consideration is to see how the posing of the question directs the entire EBT process.

Example 2:
P = students in the clinical setting
S = simulation experiences
C = experiences with actual clients
O = improved perception of clinical principles
T = (none used)

As these aspects are composed into a question format, the resulting question emerges: Do students who use simulation experiences in place of clinical experiences with actual clients exhibit improved knowledge of clinical principles within the clinical setting?

A third example of the use of the PSCOT format to determine the best practices available in the learning environment is as follows.

Example 3:
P = students between the ages of 18 to 45
S = delivery of course materials via an online hybrid course-delivery method
C = delivery of course materials via face-to-face active participation course-delivery method
O = increased comprehension of course material
T = (none used)

Taking these components to direct the inquiry into the investigation of the evidence would result in the question: Do students between the ages of 18 to 45 have increased comprehension of course material when the material is delivered by an online hybrid method in comparison to a face-to-face active participation format? A final example of the development of EBT questions is as follows.

Example 4:
P = novice faculty
S = use of designated preceptors
C = use of scheduled faculty development sessions
O = increased ease in managing the role
T = following the first year of practice

When using these concepts to formulate a question to investigate, the question could be worded as: Do novice faculty members who have a designated preceptor compared to the use of scheduled faculty development sessions during the first year of working as a faculty member have an increased ease in the performance of the faculty role?

Once the question has been determined, the process of EBT continues with the investigation into the evidence (Table 1-2). The exploring of the evidence results from the key concepts and facets identified within the question. Each of the different pieces of the puzzle is used to distinguish the strategic articles and data which can be used to support and/or negate the educational strategy under scrutiny. The discovery and analysis of the articles and data can take many different forms but must address the gaps and/or consistencies within the information available in relation to the teaching strategy.

As the articles and data are summarized to provide a clear and concise picture of the evidence that is accessible related to the topic, the process of EBT necessitates that the students' characteristics, preferences, and values be considered at this point. Though EBT and EBP utilize the evidence as the foundation for practice, the characteristics, preferences, and values of the participants must also be considered as plans for the next phases of the process are considered. Damron-Rodriquez (2008) acknowledged that the three stages within the "knowledge transfer framework" are: "knowledge is created and distilled, then it is diffused and disseminated, and finally it is adopted, implemented, and institutionalized" (p. 41). The knowledge transfer framework is supported and utilized by the Agency of Healthcare Research and Quality (AHRQ). Evidence is critical but must be balanced by the individualization of the process for the unique setting in which the teaching strategy is to be used.

After carefully composing the question, investigating the evidence, and considering the uniqueness of the participants, the process of EBT challenges the members involved to integrate academic, financial, and resource boundaries into the plan for utilization of best practices. As opportunities to use the optimum teaching strategy in an educational setting are determined, each of these facets (students, academic environment, financial, and resources) must be conscientiously considered and integrated to ensure that the final outcome is effective. Within the educational environment, it is ill advised to plan changes without considering the financial boundaries, resource availability, student population, and academic environment. Each educational institution is unique and must be considered within the plans to incorporate changes in the learning process based upon the evidence.

The final aspect within EBT is the evaluation of the process. For each question and consideration, key performance criteria must be used to determine if the process and the changes are facilitating the learning within a particular environment. The PSCOT has outcomes listed. These outcomes reflect performance criteria that can be used to further advance the evidence related to the educational strategy under consideration. According to Adams and Valiga (2009), "excellence is the kind of thing 'we know when we see it,' but defining it accurately is very difficult" (p. 3). Coming to an understanding of how to effectively apply EBP principles to the teaching/learning environment requires succinct and straightforward thinking by leaders in the educational community. Adams and Valiga (2009) further state that "it means setting high standards for yourself and the group in which you are involved, holding yourself to those standards despite challenges or pressures to reduce or lower them, and not being satisfied with anything less that the very best" (p. 3). Just like nurses had to step up to the plate and accept the principles of EBP, nursing educators must delve into the abyss to organize and establish the concepts and measures imperative for EBT. The advancement of the nursing educational environment requires that each member accept the responsibility of holding fast to high standards. A key approach that will allow the establishment and maintenance of high standards is the confirmation of the teaching/learning aspects though sound and effective evidence.

Critical Thinking

When discussing EBP and EBT definitions and steps, one essential requirement is consideration of the connection of critical thinking to EBP and EBT. Achieving positive patient outcomes requires faculty who think critically about how and what they teach and students who can take content and apply it to practice through critical thinking. Before going further, perhaps an understanding of critical thinking is necessary.

Paul, Elder, and Bartell (1997) indicate that the origin of critical thinking began 2500 years ago in the time of Socrates and has gained momentum over the years. In 2005, Fitzpatrick suggested nursing, as a discipline, was influenced by David Schron in his classic 1983 work. Ard (2009) also suggested that critical thinking isn't new, and since the 1990s, many publications about critical thinking have emerged. Multiple organizations, such as the AACN, the NLN, and even the Institute of Medicine (IOM), have emphasized the importance of the teaching and application of critical thinking in the provision of patient care. As a result, the subject of critical thinking is a major topic, and "critical thinking" has become a common buzzword in education and practice.

The current emphasis surrounding critical thinking has generated two major controversies related to critical thinking. The first controversy centers on the definition of critical thinking. Thompson (2009), Webber (2008), and Birx (2006) all suggest there is no common standard definition of critical thinking in nursing. The lack of a clear definition leads one to question: If we don't know what it is, then how can we do it? If critical thinking is essential to providing nursing care, how can we translate it into practice? It is beyond the scope of this book to offer all aspects and definitions of critical thinking, but a review of several definitions will provide insight, terms, and an applicable definition for use in EBT.

In 1987, Ennis defined critical thinking as "reasonable reflective thinking that is focused on deciding what to believe or do" (p. 10). Birx (2006) suggests that Paul and Nosich's 1991 definition is more commonly accepted: "Critical thinking is the intellectually disciplined process of actively and skillfully conceptualizing, applying, analyzing, synthesizing, and evaluating information gathered from or generated by observation, experience, reflecting, reasoning, or communication, as a guide to belief or action" (p. 4, p. 300). Paul (2004) suggests that critical thinking is an art that involves analyzing and assessing thinking to get to a better process of thinking.

Terms often associated with critical thinking in nursing include the nursing process, problem solving, rational approach, decision making, reflection, concept mapping, and evidence such as scientific research. The terms have relevance to defining critical thinking. For the purpose of this textbook, critical thinking will be defined as the art of analyzing and applying information gathered to make decisions regarding nursing care.

The second controversy involves whether or not critical thinking can be taught. Paul (2004) states that studies indicate faculty do not understand the concept of critical thinking, and faculty teach content such as math or biology but not mathematical or biological thinking. At an AACN business meeting in 2009, Bain (2009) indicated that Dewey suggested people don't learn by experience but rather by thinking about experience. Hesslip (1993, 2008) goes further to say that a professional nurse must think like a nurse, which is different from the perspective of a doctor or other health professional concerning how the patient is viewed and the problems associated with providing nursing care. Thus, nurses reason differently than other healthcare providers and nursing faculty need to teach nursing thinking. Perhaps an example of a clinical learning situation might provide insight into how you would approach critical thinking. A fourth-semester senior student just approached you and said, "My patient is complaining of pain in her arm where I just started an IV. I don't think I hurt her. What should I do?" How would you teach the student to critically think about the situation? Would you tell her what to do? Would you just take care of the problem and then discuss what you did and why? Is your approach a way to teach nursing thinking?

Assessing Sources of Evidence-Based Teaching

According to Oermann (2009), "without research and other types of evidence, decisions are often made by the most vocal faculty members, for expediency, or in response to a pressing need" (p. 64). How sad it is that nursing education bows to the most vocal faculty members rather than seeking and utilizing an EBT approach. As the expectation for state-of-the-art teaching/learning strategies becomes increasingly accepted and expected, the need to access the literature to find the current data becomes of principal importance.

Nursing faculty members must ensure that they are information literate. *Information literacy* is defined by the American Library Association (2006) as "a set of abilities requiring individuals to recognize when information is needed and have the ability to locate, evaluate, and use effectively the needed information" ("What Is Information Literacy," bullet 1). Two key databases that can be used are CINAHL (the database of nursing and allied health literature) and PubMed (the National Library of Medicine's bibliographic database). Both of these databases index any published studies related to nursing education. Since EBT is a new area, a further investigation into the educational databases of Education Resources Information (ERIC), PsycINFO, and other databases specific to any question posed should be conducted.

When selecting a database, it is helpful to understand that databases can follow one of two structures. Some databases are set up as bibliographic databases. This type of database provides information about the publication such as author, title, journal name, or publisher. Within a bibliographic database, abstracts and/or synopses are available for review. The second type of structure for databases is the full-text format. Within this format, the database allows access to the whole article. Thus, an individual can view the text, charts, graphs, references, and so forth.

Another important aspect within information literacy is to understand that databases have languages unique to their materials. A database will either have a specific controlled vocabulary (thesaurus) or use the MeSH headings. The MeSH headings are those headings established by the National Library of Medicine's thesaurus for MEDLINE. The MeSH headings can be accessed through www.nlm.nih.gov/mesh/meshhome.html. By using the MeSH headings to direct the literature review, the number of articles can be streamlined to a more manageable level. These headings and/or other keys derived from the PSCOT help to narrow the focus and get at the appropriate articles within the literature, thus saving time and energy by not accessing ineffective articles.

Only by using healthcare, educational, and other specific databases to query the literature can a full understanding of the current state of a teaching/learning strategy be understood. It is imperative when conducting a literature search that multiple databases be utilized to ensure that the subject has been addressed from multiple directions. By using this approach, the strength of the search is improved.

As articles and evidence are located within the databases and other sites, an evaluation of the information located must be tempered by the nurse educator's specific educational setting. The rating and scoring of evidence related to the applicability is of prime importance. Several organizations have evidence-rating mechanisms available to use within this process. The Cochrane Collaboration, AHRQ, and multiple textbooks provide examples of the different rating mechanisms. Though these rating mechanisms provide a means for evaluating the literature, each instructor must also gauge the literature within the specific context of the educational setting. The instructor must weigh the evidence to determine if it answers the PSCOT question posed and whether it is applicable to the specific setting. The application to a specific setting is unique to the setting. Each faculty member must accept the responsibility of determining if the evidence is relevant in a particular setting. Oermann (2009) correctly states that "our problem is not a lack of innovation in nursing education, but instead a lack of evidence about those innovations" (p. 74). Faculty members must take on the challenge of moving the preliminary studies into the next level, where fully developed studies in a larger controlled setting are conducted and disseminated. McCartney and Morin (2005) support this idea by stating that knowledge of the science of education is fundamental to improve the achievements of the individual both as a teacher and as a facilitator of learning for the students.

Critically Appraising Knowledge for Teaching Decision Making

Finding and assessing sources of EBT leads faculty to ask: How do I decide what needs to be taught? Although there may be a paucity of literature on EBT, the current explosion of information, regardless of content for any nursing course, can be overwhelming. Faculty members have a prescribed amount of time to teach a course. As a result, faculty cohorts have to sift through mountains of material and decide what must be taught versus what would be nice or great to teach. Once again, critical thinking must occur, but this time the faculty members aren't teaching critical thinking, but rather applying critical thinking regarding the selection of content that will adequately supply knowledge about a given subject. Perhaps using the "see one, do one, teach one" phrase has application to the decisions faculty must make regarding the content to be taught. Through continuing nursing education and formal education programs, faculty members have seen other educators presenting content. Faculty can draw upon those experiences by thinking about how the educators in their experience assembled the content to be taught. Having seen items such as outlines, handouts, references, and all the multiple instructional aids, faculty can begin to see how content is selected, organized, and presented. Care must be taken to ensure that the educator is skilled. Another caution, at this point, is that always teaching the way you were taught may not be EBT.

Once again, faculty members need to turn to the literature. By using the methods for assessing courses as previously discussed, faculty members can then begin to cull through the content to be taught. Other aspects will play a major role in appraising knowledge for making decisions about what to teach. Program, curriculum, and evaluation design, teaching/learning strategies, licensure examinations, and accreditation are just a few considerations that will influence content and will be discussed in future chapters.

Summary Thoughts

Evidence-based practice and evidence-based teaching go hand in hand with critical thinking. The emergence of EBP and now EBT has provided an educational environment that promotes critical thinking for both faculty and students. The steps of EBP and EBT are foundational to critical thinking about the sources of EBT and the selection of content to be presented.

Summary Points

1. Scholarship in EBT advances the development of the art and science of nursing education.
2. Several models of EBP have emerged since the 1970s.
3. Multiple definitions of EBP exist but definitions for EBT are few in number.
4. EBT is defined as a dynamic, holistic system using educational principles validated by evidence to support, maintain, and promote a new level of knowledge for a learner in a variety of settings.
5. The steps of EBP have application to EBT.
6. To structure an EBT question, the format should include population, strategy, comparison, outcome, and time (PSCOT).
7. Critical thinking is much discussed but two major controversies exist: what is critical thinking, and can it be taught?
8. Assessing sources of EBT requires faculty to be informed about literature databases.
9. Critically appraising knowledge for making decisions for teaching involves EBP, EBT, and critical thinking.

Tips for Nurse Educators to Use

1. Be knowledgeable about EBP and EBT in relation to definitions, steps, similarities, and differences.
2. Explore your own values regarding what critical thinking is and whether you believe it can be taught.
3. Connect with a librarian to obtain current, accurate sources for EBT.
4. Identify how you critically appraise content to be taught.

References

Adams, M. H., & Valiga, T. M. (2009). *Achieving excellence in nursing education.* New York, NY: National League for Nursing.

American Association of Colleges of Nursing. (1999). Position statement on defining scholarship for the discipline of nursing. Retrieved October 8, 2009, from www.aacn.nche.edu/Publications/positions/scholar.htm

American Library Association. (2006). Information literacy competency standards for higher education. Retrieved November 1, 2009, from www.ala.org/ala/mgrps/divs/acrl/standards/informationliteracycompetency.cfm

Appling, S. E., Naumann, P. L., & Berk, R. A. (2001). Using a faculty evaluation triad to achieve evidence-based teaching. *Nursing & Health Care Perspectives,* 22(5), 247–251.

Ard, N. (2009). Essentials of learning. In Cathleen M. Schultz (Ed.), *Essentials of learning in building a science of nursing education: Foundation for evidence-based teaching learning.* New York, NY: National League for Nursing.

Bain, K. (2009). Personal communication. American Association of College of Nursing Business meeting, November 1, 2009, Washington, DC.

Birx, E. C. (2006). Critical thinking and theory based practice. In W. K. Cody (Ed.), *Philosophical and theoretical perspectives for advanced nursing practice.* Sudbury, MA: Jones and Bartlett Publishers.

Boswell, C., & Cannon, S. (2011). *Introduction to nursing research: Incorporating evidence-based practice* (2nd ed.). Sudbury, MA: Jones & Bartlett Publishers.

Boyer, E. L. (1990). *Scholarship reconsidered: Priorities of the professoriate.* New York, NY: The Carnegie Foundation for the Advancement of Teaching.

Damron-Rodriquez, J. (2008). Developing competence for nurses and social workers. *American Journal of Nursing,* 108(9 Supplement), 40–46.

Danielson, C. (2008). *Handbook for enhancing professional practice: Evidence of teaching.* Association for Supervision and Curriculum Development. Retrieved August 13, 2009, from www.ascd.org/publications/books/106035/chapters/Evidence_of_Teaching.aspx

Emerson, R. J., & Records, K. (2008). Today's challenge, tomorrow's excellence: The practice of evidence-based education. *Journal of Nursing Education,* 47(8), 359–370.

Ennis, R. H. (1987). A taxonomy of critical thinking dispositions and abilities. In J. B. Baron & R. J. Sternberg (Eds.), *Teaching thinking skill: Theory and practice.* New York, NY: W.H. Fresynk.

Fitzpatrick, J. (2005). Critical thinking: How do we know it in nursing education and practice? *Nursing Education Perspective,* 26(5), 261.

Hesslip. P. (1993, revised 2008). Critical thinking: To think like a nurse. Retrieved October 25, 2009, from www.criticalthinking.org/resources/HE/ctandnursing.cfm

Magee, M. (2005). *Health politics: Power, population, and health.* Bronxville, NY: Spencer Books.

Malloch, K., & Porter-O'Grady, (2006). *Introduction to evidence-based practice in nursing and health care.* Sudbury, MA: Jones and Bartlett Publishers.

McCartney, P. R., & Morin, K. H. (2005). Where is the evidence for teaching methods used in nursing education? *The American Journal of Maternal Child Nursing,* 30(6), 406–412.

Melnyk, B. M., & Fineout-Overholt, E. (2005). *Evidence-based practice in nursing and healthcare: A guide to best practice.* Philadelphia, PA: Lippincott Williams & Wilkins.

Oermann, M. H. (2009). Evidence-based programs and teaching/evaluation methods: Needed to achieve excellence in nursing education. In M. H. Adams & T. M. Valiga (Eds.), *Achieving excellence in nursing education* (Chapter 6) New York, NY: National League for Nursing.

Paul, R. (2004). The state of critical thinking today. Retrieved October 25, 2009, from www.criticalthinking.org/professionalDEV/The_state_ct_today.cfm

Paul, R., Elder, L., & Bartell, T. (1997). Taken from the California teacher preparation for instruction in critical thinking: Research findings and policy recommendations. State of California, California Commission on Teacher Credentialing, Sacramento, CA. Retrieved October 25, 2009, from www.criticalthinking.org/aboutCT/briefHistoryCT.cfm

Porter-O'Grady, T. (2006). A new age for practice: Creating the framework for evidence. In K. Malloch & T. Porter-O'Grady (Eds.), *Introduction to evidence-based practice in nursing and health care.* Sudbury, MA: Jones and Bartlett Publishers.

Pravikoff, D. S., Tanner, A. B., & Pierce, S. T. (2005). Readiness of U.S. nurses for evidence-based practice. *American Journal of Nursing, 105*(9), 40–51.

Rutledge, D. N., & Grant, M. (2002). Introduction. *Seminars in Oncology Nursing, 18,* 1–2.

Shultz, C. M. (2009). *Building a science of nursing education: Foundation for evidence-based teaching-learning.* New York, NY; National League for Nursing.

Thompson, C. (2009). Teaching-learning in the cognitive domain. In C. M. Schultz (Ed.), *Essentials of learning in building a science of nursing education: Foundation for evidence-based teaching learning.* New York, NY: National League for Nursing.

Webber, P. B. (2008). Facilitating critical thinking and effective reasoning. In B. K. Penn (Ed.), *Mastering the teaching role: A guide for nurse educators.* Philadelphia, PA: F.A. Davis Company.

Webster's II New College Dictionary. (1995). Orlando, FL: Houghton Mifflin.

Wexler, J. M. (n.d.). Evidence-based teaching at Dartmouth: Students helping teachers. Retrieved October 9, 2009, from www.dartmouth.edu/~thepress/read.php?id=1352

Web Links

MeSH headings can be accessed through www.nlm.nih.gov/mesh/meshhome.html. The National League for Nursing (NLN) Excellence in Nursing Education Model is viewable at www.nln.org/excellence/model/index.htm.

Multiple Choice Questions

1. The initial Evidence-based Practice method resulted in the development of the

    A. ARCC.

    B. Cochrane Center/Collaboration.

    C. Joanne Briggs Institute.

    D. Rosswurn-Larrabee model.

Rationale:

As a result of Cochrane's pioneering work in 1972, the Cochrane Center in Oxford, England, was established in 1992 and the Cochrane Collaboration was recognized in 1993. The premise for the Cochrane Collaboration is to advance healthcare decision making through the use of systematic reviews concerning the outcome evidence from healthcare interventions. The Cochrane Collaboration and Center are international, not-for-profit, independent organizations that are committed to ensuring that state-of-the-art, accurate information concerning the outcomes of healthcare interventions is accessible by the global community.

2. One area *not* seen in the characteristics of EBP is

    A. provider expertise.

    B. client contribution.

    C. cost.

    D. decision-making scheme.

Rationale:

According to Boswell and Cannon (2011), the constant characteristics which are found within the multiple definitions are the decision-making scheme, clinical application, provider expertise, and client contribution.

3. A systems approach is understood to include

    A. interrelated, interacting, and/or interdependent constituents.

    B. unit-specific constituents.

    C. unilateral, reactive, and/or interdependent constituents.

    D. global, specific constituents.

Rationale:

The EBP process is viewed within a systems approach, and a "system is viewed as a group of interrelated, interacting, and/or interdependent constituents forming a complex whole" (*Webster's II New College Dictionary*, 1995, p. 1119).

4. The PSCOT format for developing an EBT statement represents

    A. problem, situation, cost, outcome, time.

    B. problem, strategy, comparison, outcome, time.

C. population, situation, comparison, outcome, target.

D. population, strategy, comparison, outcome, time.

Rationale:

The "P" represents the population. The population within the educational process can be directed toward students, administrators, faculty, alumni, candidates, preceptors, coaches, and many other groups of individuals who are involved in the educational process. The "S" represents the educational strategy. Educational strategies are any aspect within the educational environment that comes into play for advancing the success of the learning process. The "C" within the format mirrors the "C" within the EBP format. The incorporation of a comparison of educational strategies provides an evaluation of the different avenues for advancing the learning environment. The "O" within the format also parallels the inclusion of outcome as used in the EBP format. The final aspect, the "T," is the incorporation of the time period when applicable.

5. In what manner is EBP different from EBT?

   A. Evidence-based practice focuses on the clinical setting.
   B. Evidence-based teaching focuses on the educational setting.
   C. Evidence-based practice includes only research results.
   D. Evidence-based teaching is no different that evidence-based practice.

Rationale:

Whereas EBP works within the clinical realm, EBT resides within a multiplicity of settings, which can include the clinical realm.

6. Two key databases for use during the literature review are:

   A. CINAHL and ERIC.
   B. CINAHL and PubMed.
   C. PubMed and ERIC.
   D. PubMed and Google.

Rationale:

The two key databases are CINAHL (the database of nursing and allied health literature) and PubMed (the National Library of Medicine's bibliographic database).

7. The critical step required to be successful in conducting EBT is

   A. conducting a thorough literature review.
   B. always including a comparison and intervention.
   C. establishing the student preferences.
   D. posing an effective question.

Rationale:

The posing of the question is the crucial initial step for the initiation of an investigation into the evidence surrounding the educational process. The wording of the question must be clear and concise.

8. The initial step used when conducting a literature review is:
   A. pulling all of the articles that can be located on the topic.
   B. selecting appropriate terms, such as MeSH terms, related to the topic.
   C. omitting all articles older than 5 years.
   D. selecting only articles that are research based.

Rationale:

A database will either have a specific controlled vocabulary (thesaurus) or use the MeSH headings. The MeSH headings are those headings established by the National Library of Medicine's thesaurus for MEDLINE. By using the MeSH headings to direct the literature review, the number of articles can be streamlined to a more manageable level.

9. Critical thinking in nursing can be defined as
   A. the science of teaching ways of thinking about nursing care.
   B. the art of analyzing and applying information gathered to make decisions regarding nursing care.
   C. a method of making decisions about nursing care.
   D. the systematic process of thinking that results in optimal patient outcomes.

Rationale:

For the purpose of this textbook, critical thinking is defined as the art of analyzing and applying information gathered to make decisions regarding nursing care.

10. The current knowledge explosion in health care
    A. impacts what is taught in nursing courses.
    B. makes selection of course content easier.
    C. allows faculty to quickly decide content to be taught.
    D. is not a problem for determining course content.

Rationale:

As a result of the knowledge explosion, faculty members have to sift through mountains of material and decide what must be taught versus what would be nice or great to teach. Once again, critical thinking must occur, but this time the faculty members aren't teaching critical thinking but rather applying critical thinking regarding the selection of content that will adequately supply knowledge about a given subject.

11. The center of the process within EBT is the

    A. client.

    B. faculty member.

    C. student.

    D. school process.

Rationale:

The learner is viewed as the center of the process within EBT. It is within the learner that each and every educational session and resource intermingles to ensure that the learner is effectively placed in a position to gain the utmost knowledge from the educational environment.

12. A well-developed PSCOT question provides the focus for

    A. selection of key words and concepts used to narrow the determination of the articles.

    B. selection of articles based on the population and outcomes.

    C. directing of the literature search by identifying selected articles.

    D. management of the EBP process outside of the educational focus.

Rationale:

A well-developed question provides the key words and concepts imperative for identifying and narrowing the selection of the articles. By successfully ascertaining the articles through the literature search driven by the question, evidence that supports the teaching environment can be discovered.

Discussion Questions

1. You have been assigned to teach nursing theories in a 6-week online course. How will you approach the selection of content to be taught?

Considerations:

■ How many nursing theories exist? Which theories are most commonly used?

■ Determine the reading assignments and coursework students must be able to complete each week.

■ Assign a group or individual students to a theorist to report back on a discussion board.

2. As you begin to mentor a novice faculty member, the individual asks for help in determining the best way to facilitate a fundamental clinical group of 10 students. Formulate a PSCOT question and determine the key words to use for a literature review as you demonstrate EBT to this individual.

Considerations:

■ PSCOT–population, strategy, comparison, outcome, time

■ Key terms should reflect MeSH terms

3. Identify one example of evidence that is available for:

    a. A teaching strategy that you are comfortable using.

    b. A teaching strategy that was regularly used when you were a student.

    c. A teaching strategy that you are considering using.

Considerations:

■ Formulate PSCOT question.

■ Pull key words using MeSH terms.

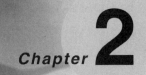

Chapter 2

The Role of the Academician

Sharon Cannon and Carol Boswell

Chapter Objectives

At the conclusion of this chapter, the learner will be able to:

1. Discuss generational differences as they apply to the educational experience.
2. Determine a plan for managing generational aspects within the academician's role.
3. Examine curricular issues using an evidence-based teaching approach.
4. Contrast the role of the academician in relation to committee involvement.
5. Compare key issues related to tenure and promotion within the educational experience.
6. Discuss the expectation and value of evidence-based teaching policies and procedures.

Key Terms

➤ Academician

➤ Baby Boomers

➤ Committee

➤ Contextual learning

➤ Curriculum

➤ Directive learning

➤ Generation X

➤ Generational cohort

➤ Hard skills

➤ Inquiry learning

➤ Item learning

➤ Millennials

➤ Mission

➤ Philosophy

➤ Policy

➤ Procedure

➤ Promotion

➤ Rational learning

➤ Soft skills

➤ Syntactical learning

➤ Tenure

➤ Veterans

Introduction

As faculty members begin to acknowledge the need for evidence-based teaching (EBT), several concepts related to the academician's role must be carefully considered and incorporated. Never before in history has the workplace been required to engage four distinct generational cohorts. Sherman (2006) defines a **generational cohort** as "a group of people who share birth years, history, and a collective personality as a result of their defining experiences" (p. 2). As with any grouping of individuals, the group members may display many of the same characteristics but individuals will also have unique characteristics. The information available about generational groups is founded on research evidence as well as opinion evidence. Most of the work has been completed outside of the profession of nursing but is valid when considering the different characteristics of the cohorts. Faculty members must take care that while considering the characteristics for the generational cohort, they do not lose sight that each student and faculty member is also a result of his or her unique heritage. The four cohorts currently present in the workplace are: the **Veterans**, the **Baby Boomers**, **Generation X**, and the **Millennials** (Hahn, 2009; Wieck, 2008). Hahn (2009) states "the challenge for the nurse manager is to embrace and respect the multigenerational diversity of the staff while developing and supporting a highly functioning and cohesive nursing team" (p. 8). Though this idea is true for the nurse manager, it is equally true for the educator. The educator frequently represents either the Veterans or Baby Boomer cohort but must educate the Generation X and Millennial cohorts. We are seeing the Generation X cohort beginning to step up to the plate and assume the educator role. As a result, we have educators potentially from three different cohorts. Although the students may be from numerous generational groups (e.g., Silent Generation, Baby Boomers, Generation X, or Millennial), the student cohorts tend to be primarily from either the Generation X or Millennial groups. The Silent Generation is those individuals who are seen as having years of experience who are approaching or engaged in retirement at this point in their lives. Thus, the faculty cohort may be dealing with the challenge of embracing and respecting these different generational needs within the faculty group in addition to the management of the Generation X and Millennials within the classroom.

According to Wieck (2008), "Millennial youngsters are the best educated, most affluent and most ethnically diverse of the four generations in the workplace today" (p. 27). This group of individuals values education but not necessarily in the same manner that the Veterans and Baby Boomer groups do. How each of the generational distinctions comes to bear on the academician's role provides many challenges. The faculty members must carefully engage in productive management of the educational environment based on these different generational characteristics as they address the academic issues of curriculum, committee involvement, tenure and promotion issues, and policy and procedure development. An effective faculty body will use the strengths and manage the weaknesses from each of these generational cohorts to develop and manage an educational program which is visionary and strategically savvy.

Generational Aspects for Both Faculty and Students

The majority of the information available within the nursing literature concerning the generational differences is directed toward the management of the workplace. Thus, educators must take the information provided and apply it to the educational experience. Hammill (2005) states that "roles today are all over the place and the rules are being rewritten daily" (p. 2). As nursing faculty members, we are called upon to correlate information found in one area with how it applies to another area. Hammill (2005) goes on to state that generational dissimilarities can influence everything from recruiting, fostering teams, and managing change, to encouraging, overseeing, and developing efficiency and output. These same areas are key aspects within the educational environment. Faculty members must develop a sound foundational knowledge about generational strengths and challenges to ensure the success of the educational process while decreasing the frustrations that emerge when conflict and stress are present. Taking the time and energy to consider the different generations and work to meet them somewhere in the middle can and will improve the educational outcomes for a program.

The evidence presented in **Table 2-1** provides a starting point for investigating generational characteristics that can be used to formulate a functional faculty cohort that can effectively work with the

Table 2-1

General Generational Characteristics			
Veterans (born before 1945)	**Baby Boomers (born 1946–1964)**	**Generation X (born 1965–1976)**	**Millennials (born 1977–1997)**
Generational Values • Hard working • Respect for authority • Disciplined • Accept delayed rewards • Adhere to rules • Conformers • Dedication/ sacrifice • Duty before pleasure • Trust in government	• Optimistic • Team players • Strong work effort • Personal gratification • Anything is possible • Want to "make a difference"	• Diverse • Self-reliant • Free agents • Balanced • Informal • Fun • Highly educated • Think globally • Techno literacy	• Globally diverse • Optimistic • Achievement oriented • Flexible • Avid consumers • Civic duty • Extreme fun • Hotly competitive • Street smarts • Realism • Extremely techno savvy
Generational Strengths • Stable • Detail oriented • Loyal • Hard working • Reliable • Practical • Dedicated • Ethical • Fiscally prudent • Honorable • Task oriented • Follow rules of conduct	• Driven • Team, service, and relationship oriented • Optimistic • Have ability to handle a crisis • Ambitious • Ethical • Have good communication skills • Live to work • Multitaskers • Politically correct	• Accepting of change • Capable of multitasking • Technologically literate • Self-reliant • Creative • Skeptical • Balanced • Self-starters • Results driven • Self-sufficient • Work to live	• Optimistic • Capable of multitasking • Very technologically savvy • Outcome driven • Determined • Ambitious but not entirely focused • Best educated– confident • Open to new ideas • Self-absorbed • Respect given for competency not title
Other Names Traditionalists, Silent Generation, Moral Authority, The Forgotten Generation	"Me" Generation, Moral Authority	Gen X, Xers, The Doers, Post Boomers, 13th Generation, Busters, Twenty Somethings	Generation Y, Gen Y, Generation Next, Echo Boomers, Chief Friendship Officers, 24/7 Bridgers, Mosaics, Net Generation

Source: Adapted from Hahn, J. (2009). Effectively manage a multigenerational staff. *Nursing Management, 40*(9), 8–10; http://www.wmfc.org/GenerationalDifferencesChart.pdf; and Gaylor, D. (2002). Generational differences. Retrieved November 24, 2009, from http://www.reachtheu.com.

differences encountered. Within this table, the values and strengths for each of the four generations are provided for comparison along with the numerous titles that can be used within the literature to depict the different generational divisions. The division within the work environment is depicted to be approximately 5% Veterans, 45% Baby Boomers, 40% Generation Xers, and 10% Millennials. Several key aspects in regard to the values are evident. The Generation X and Millennial generations are considered to be technologically literate. Since technology is very important to these two generations, the educational environment must embrace and assimilate technology into the classroom and clinical experience. The differences and similarities between each of the generations should be carefully considered. The Baby Boomers are optimistic but desire personal gratification. Generation X, on the other hand, is informal and diverse. The Baby Boomers, though wanting to make a difference, are expecting that their generation will be the group to address the challenges confronting the educational and workplace environment. Generation X wants to enjoy the world while considering themselves as free agents who are self-reliant. The Millennial generation explodes onto the educational and workplace environments with a fun-loving attitude as well as civic-mindedness. Work is considered to be a requirement by this group but must be confronted in a realistic and ambitious manner. As faculty members consider each of these aspects, one area to conscientiously evaluate is the need to restructure the course delivery to embrace the openness, civic focus, and self-reliant aspects within these groups.

Within **Table 2-2**, the focus for each generation related to engagement with others is presented and reflects the evidence as currently understood. The perception of the Millennial generation concerning education being extremely expensive is cause for concern. Faculty members must remember this perception and ensure that the majority of the educational process is viewed as realistic and meaningful. Since the idea is that education is costly, the practicality of the material presented is imperative. Another dimension important for the faculty to commit to memory is the value for each of the two generations: Generation X (Gen X) looks at the time commitment of the experience whereas the Millennials desire the uniqueness of the experience. So often, the phase "Tell me what I need to know for the test" is identified as an expectation from students. With the understanding of the focus for these two groups, the rationale for this statement can be better understood. Faculty members must consider the time commitment and the uniqueness of each encounter within the educational process. Clear delineation as to the rationale for each experience needs to be addressed, thus providing value for the encounter. Another primary area resulting in stress and frustration as the generations come

Table 2-2

Generational Characteristics and Work-Related Aspects

	Veterans (born before 1945)	Baby Boomers (born 1946–1964)	Generation X (born 1965–1976)	Millennials (born 1977–1997)
Education	An aspiration	A birthright	A means to progress forward	A staggering expense
Value	Family/community	Achievement	Time	Uniqueness
Focus	Duty	Associations and outcome	Tasks and outcome	International and networked
Interactive Style	Individual	Team player Revere meetings	Entrepreneur	Participative
View on Respect for Authority	Authority is based on seniority and tenure	Skeptical of authority Time equals authority	Skeptical of authority figures, Will test authority repetitively	Test authority but seek out authority figures when looking for guidance
Work Ethics That Impact Educational Process	Adhere to rules Responsibility before fun Expect everyone to honor commitments Expect to be respected Linear Word is their bond Value honor, due process, fair play, good attitude, hard work, attendance	Confront authority Abhor conformity and rules Loyal to team members Process oriented Endeavor to do very best Willing to take risks Work efficiently Demand respect from younger individuals Value teamwork, personal fulfillment, equality, collaboration	Expect to influence the terms and conditions Work/family balance important Like a casual environment Outcome oriented Output focused Prefer diversity, technology, informality, and fun Want to get in, get the work done, and move on to other things	Believe (due to technology) they can work flexibly anytime, anyplace Evaluated on work product, not how, when, or where done High expectations of leaders to mentor them toward attainment of goals Goal oriented Mentoring is important Obsessed with career development Tolerant Thrive in a collaborative environment Seek continuing education to enhance work skills

Source: Adapted from Hahn, J. (2009). Effectively manage a multigenerational staff. *Nursing Management, 40*(9), 8–10; http://www.wmfc.org/GenerationalDifferencesChart.pdf; and Gaylor, D. (2002). Generational differences. Retrieved November 24, 2009, from http://www.reachtheu.com.

together is the differing views on respect for authority. Both Gen Xers and Millennials expect to test authority repeatedly. Millennials differ in that while testing the authority figure, they continue to seek guidance from that authority. In contrast, the idea held by the Baby Boomers concerning the importance of time in establishment of the authority can result in stress. Baby Boomers perceive that a person with time and experience should be identified as having authority.

Gen Xers and Millennials do not see time involved as a foundation for authority. The amount of time that a person works at a job does not equate to the person having the authority to manage a position per the Gen X and Millennial cohorts. Faculty members must understand that from these generations' viewpoint, being a nurse for multiple years does not mean that the person is, nor can be, an effective teacher. Gen Xers and Millennials seek to find individuals who have the experience but also knowledge about how to get a message across. These individuals are the ones that the Gen Xers and Millennial cohorts will embrace as having authority. In addition to the thoughts about authority, an additional difference between the Gen Xers and Millennial cohorts is based on the viewpoint of work ethics. In Table 2-2, some of the different work ethics are listed. Gen Xers are focused on self, whereas Millennials embrace the idea of mentorship. Millennials value involvement with authorities, whereas Gen Xers seem to prefer doing things alone. In regard to work ethics, Gen Xers seem to want to be told what to do by the leader, then the leader needs to step back and let them do it their way. Although the Millennials want to be allowed to do it their way, they seek mentors to help them to work it out. They also want to select their own mentors based on who they perceive as having authority, not by who has a title.

As faculty members strive to engage the different generations in the learning process, several additional ideas need to be considered (**Table 2-3**). The Millennial (Gen Y) cohort treasures the ability to work with bright and energetic individuals. Faculty members coming to the work environment excited about the opportunities and challenges are means for connecting with this generational group. Gen Xers, on the other hand, appreciate freedom to approach problems and challenges in unique ways. Rules are not appreciated by this generation because many regulations are based upon the here and now. Gen Xers view the application of rules and regulations as frequently contingent on the current environment. Gen Xers view these changing practices as fluid and not set in stone. Thus, freedom to investigate innovative ways to address the challenge and/or problem is a mainstay within the expectations for the Gen Xers population. Faculty members who primarily are within the Baby Boomers group desire that their wisdom and experience be valued and accepted when challenges and problems are identified. The tested ways are embraced by the Baby Boomers, whereas an open slate for managing the issues is celebrated by the Gen Xers group. Baby Boomer faculty members must allow the Gen Xers group to try out new approaches while respecting the teamwork orientation found within the Millennials. Gen X individuals do not like teams and groups because singularity is a main principle in their value system. According to Wieck (2008), "the team orientation of the Millennials is in stark contrast to the more independent-minded

Table 2-3

Generational Work-Related Characteristics

	Veterans (born before 1945)	Baby Boomers (born 1946–1964)	Generation X (born 1965–1976)	Millennials (born 1977–1997)
Views of Authority	Respectful Endure Honor and respect	Awed Replace them Challenge leaders	Unenthusiastic Ignore leaders	Undisturbed Leaders must respect you Choose their own bosses
Role of Career	Means for living	Central focus	Irritant	Always changing
Best Ways to Interact	Know the rules and follow them Reduce the appearance of lack of discipline, respect, logic, and structure Strive to understand their feelings	Value their ideas when possible Work is important to them Silly routines are frustrating Teams Motivated by their responsibilities toward others Responsive to attention and recognition Don't take criticism well Need flexibility, attention, and freedom	Desires independence and informality Allow time to seek other interests Allow time for fun Utilize the most up-to-date technology	Use a team-oriented workplace Get to know their personal goals Treat with respect Nurtured to feel appreciated and very optimistic about self Employ appealing experiences to cultivate transferable skills Provide rationales Supply variety Grow teams and networks with immense attention Reward extra effort and excellence Provide structured, encouraging environment Utilize an interactive environment
Motivated by. . . .	Being respected Security	Being valued, needed Money	Freedom Removal of rules Time off	Working with bright people Time off

Source: Adapted from Hahn, J. (2009). Effectively manage a multigenerational staff. *Nursing Management, 40*(9), 8–10; http://www.wmfc.org/GenerationalDifferencesChart.pdf; and Gaylor, D. (2002). Generational differences. Retrieved November 24, 2009, from http://www.reachtheu.com.

Gen X" (p. 27). Millennial individuals desire teams and groups to be used to address the challenges presented in the classroom and clinical sites. Wieck (2008) continues with the idea of group engagement with the Millennial generation by stressing the importance that faculty members assign a challenge through establishing goals, forming appropriate teams, providing the teams with the freedom to address the challenge in their own ways, and ending with appropriate feedback and encouragement. One final aspect which is paramount for

Table 2-4				
Generational Characteristics—Communication and Feedback				
	Veterans (born before 1945)	**Baby Boomers (born 1946–1964)**	**Generation X (born 1965–1976)**	**Millennials (born 1977–1997)**
Communication	Discrete Present in logical manner Show respect by using titles Use formal language Don't waste time Use inclusive language (we, us) Handwritten notes More personal interaction	Diplomatic In person Direct style Present options Answer questions thoroughly Avoid manipulative/controlling language Get consensus Establish a friendly rapport	Blunt/direct Immediate Straight talk/present facts Use email as primary tool Talk in short direct phrases Share information immediately Don't micro-manage Tie the message to outcomes	Polite Positive, respectful, motivational electronic communication styles Use email and voice mail as primary tools Use action verbs Use visual pictures Be humorous Tie message to goals and aspirations
Feedback/Rewards	No news is good news Want subtle, private recognition on an individual level	Like praise and recognition Enjoy having "something for the wall" Enjoys public recognition Appreciate awards for hard work	Freedom is best reward Does not want public recognition Prefers regular feedback Needs constructive feedback	Needs frequent feedback Wants clear goals and expectations Communicate frequently
Preferred Ways to Learn Soft Skills	On the job Discussion groups Peer interaction and feedback Face-to-face coaching	On the job Discussion groups Face-to-face coaching Classroom instruction live	On the job Face-to-face coaching Assessment and feedback Discussion group	On the job Peer interaction and feedback Discussion groups Face-to-face coaching
Preferred Ways to Learn Hard Skills	Classroom instruction On the job Workbooks and manuals Books and reading	Classroom instruction On the job Workbooks and manuals Books and reading	On the job Classroom instruction Workbooks and manuals Books and reading	On the job Classroom instruction Workbooks and manuals Books and reading

Source: Adapted from Hahn, J. (2009). Effectively manage a multigenerational staff. *Nursing Management, 40*(9), 8–10; http://www.wmfc.org/GenerationalDifferencesChart.pdf; Gaylor, D. (2002). Generational differences. Retrieved November 24, 2009, from http://www.reachtheu.com and Tolbize, A. (2008). Generational differences in the workplace. *Research and Training Center on Community Living.* University of Minnesota.

the Baby Boomer faculty member to realize is the necessity for allowing time off for both the Gen Xers and Millennial groups. Both groups strongly value free, unrestricted time to embrace the world. Both the Gen Xers and Millennial cohorts expect and demand this time.

Table 2-4 provides the key areas paramount within the educational process. Communication and feedback are critical aspects of the learning process. As one compares the Baby Boomers to the Millennials, several similarities can be noted within the communication aspect. The Baby Boomers communicate with diplomacy and directness. Millennials desire communication that is polite and active in nature. Gen Xers, on the other hand, did not develop as many of the networking skills, thus they expect blunt, immediate messages. Both the Gen Xers and the Millennial generations are technologically savvy. Email and voicemail are their primary means for communication. Instant communication is highly valued. Baby Boomers and Veterans continue to value note writing and personal commitment from handwritten notes. Another interesting communication aspect is that Gen Xers want the messages tied to the outcomes, whereas Millennials value messages that are connected to the goals and aspirations. Knowledge of this message focus could be very valuable as faculty members strive to communicate with the different members within a class. Messages should be directed toward outcomes and goals/aspirations to gain support for the management of the interaction. While communicating via instant messaging, texting, and emails is of prime importance to these final two generations, it is evident that they are reading less and less. The Millennial generation strives to learn by questioning. The questions are not meant to show disrespect but to gain an understanding of how the previous generations came to the understandings that are being presented (Tolbize, 2008). This generation wants to understand the process, not just learn the facts. Millennials value instant messaging, not the reading of classics and literature. To expect them to read long assignments is beyond the custom for these groups. Another area to consider when dealing with the different generations is that of feedback and rewards. Gen Xers overall do not want public acknowledgement since they tend to be very private individuals. Feedback to this group should be regular, constructive, and allow for freedom. Millennials want frequent feedback that is tied to their focus on goals and expectations. Communication, feedback, and interactions should concentrate on management and attainment of the goals and expectations established. Faculty members would benefit by having a time at the beginning of courses for clarifying and validating the goals and expectations. For the Millennial generation, this clarification and substantiation of the goals and opportunities allows everyone to be working toward the same prize. Baby Boomers, on the other hand, desire praise and recognition. It seems that this generation values external validation, whereas the Gen X group seems to value internal validation. A final aspect to consider from a faculty member's viewpoint is the preferred routines used by the different generations for learning soft and hard skills. **Soft skills** are those activities that lend themselves to hands-on work. Each generations prefers "on-the-job" experiences when endeavoring to address these types of skills. The change comes when looking at the second way that each generation seeks to further acquire these soft skills. Both of the older generations favor the use of discussion groups as a second means of addressing the soft skills. Whereas Generation X is inclined toward face-to-face coaching as a valued process for acquiring soft skills, the Millennial group looks toward peer interaction and feedback that speaks to group encounters. In contrast, the methods desired for acquiring hard skills take different routes. **Hard skills** are those aspects that are acquired as a result of classroom experiences. Again, the older two generations desire the use of classroom instruction to develop a foundation for the hard skills, whereas both of the younger generations seek the acquisition through on-the-job training. So, basically, for both soft and hard skills, the younger generations desire the provision of the material within the job performance, or hands-on experience. As was stated previously, the younger generations do not want to be expected to read books and work on workbooks and manuals. They want to be involved with the material. O'Connor (2009) provides insight into this desire when speaking about the use of technology:

> digital literacy (adept at navigating the Web for information and are comfortable with a wide variety of technology), connected (never far from their cell phones, these learners are talking or texting constantly, including at work and in class), immediacy (expects speed and becomes impatient if they have to wait for a response or to get information), experiential (learn best by doing as opposed to being told what to do), and social team work (highly interactive and communicative). (p. 9)

Since these generations seek connectivity, faculty members must strive for ways to engage them via the Web and other immediacy types of teaching opportunities.

The technological focus embraced by both the Gen Xers and the Millennial groups is significant to the management of the classroom and clinical experience. Even during lecture and classroom activities, these groups want to be able to access the Internet to validate the material being presented and to acquire additional information that they then can share in class. O'Connor (2009) stated that "while annoying to the more mature leader and faculty member, this feeling of connectivity is of high importance to this generation" (p. 9). The ability to use technology to search the literature for evidence of clinical, management, and educational best practices is a valuable asset that the Gen Xers and Millennial groups bring to the table. This skill of the groups should be capitalized upon within the educational process and further perfected to maximize the ability to locate sound evidence on which to base practice decisions (O'Connor, 2009). The opportunities within technology to engage the students and faculty members are immeasurable when embraced.

Sherman (2006, p. 6) provides these summative recommendations for working with and among the different generations:

- Seek to understand each generational cohort.
- Accommodate generational differences in attitudes, values, and behaviors.
- Develop generationally sensitive styles to effectively coach and motivate all members of the healthcare team.
- Develop the ability to flex a communication style to accommodate generational differences.
- Promote the resolution of generational conflicts so as to build work teams.
- Capitalize on generational differences—use these differences to enhance the work of the entire team.

These simple but complex recommendations basically stem from a need to constantly be assessing our commitment to accept and engage with each generation and culture. Wieck, Dols, and Northam (2009) add to this list of recommendations with these suggestions: actively listen, give opportunities for input, build cohesive environments that are conducive to friendships, promote respectful relationships, and facilitate good communication. Each of these skills attempts to focus on the individual rather than the generational expectations. Interacting with the members of each and every generation with openness and respectfulness establishes a beginning place for the development of a sound working/learning environment. According to Tolbize (2008), "generational conflict is more likely to arise from errors of attribution and perception, than from valid differences" (p. 13). Expecting to encounter problems with the management of the generations usually always results in conflict and stress. As with working with any generation and culture, a sound knowledge of the group does help to understand when and how the group can come to the table to work and/or learn. Embracing these differences and using them to everyone's advantage allows for a "win–win" opportunity. Wieck (2008) sums it up as "The key to managing this generational mix will be open doors, open minds, and an abundance of patience" (p. 29). As we all strive to address the challenges that confront us within the academic setting, the thoughts and expectations presented by each new generation must be incorporated into our manner of delivery if we are to be successful.

Curriculum

Many different definitions can be found for the term **curriculum**. Each definition considers the idea from differing viewpoints. Oliva (1988) suggested the definition of curriculum as: "a plan or program for all the experiences which the learner encounters under the direction of the school" (p. 9). Madeus and Stufflebeam (1980) used Tanner's definition, which stated that a curriculum was the premeditated and guided learning encounters using projected learning conclusions that were devised by means of a methodical rebuilding of knowledge and experiences, within an academic setting, resulting in the learners' ongoing and deliberate evolution in personal social competence. Another example of a definition of curriculum is provided by Penn (2008) and addresses the basic components. Penn (2008) lists the components as "the mission and philosophy of the nursing unit, the conceptual framework of the program of study, course sequencing and courses required for the program of study, program objectives, learning activities, outcomes or competencies of the graduate of the program, and a program of evaluation" (p. 153). Each of these definitions implies written documents that are used to direct the learning process. Ironside (2007) takes a slightly different approach to the idea—"The most common agreement seems to be that curriculum is what actually occurs between and among persons in the educational enterprise and not some 'plan' for learning that is reflected in written materials" (p. 78). Curriculum moves from a document into a working process whereby learning can occur. The National League for Nursing established the Hallmarks of Excellence in 2004. Within the Hallmarks, the points related to curriculum are presented as (Speakman, 2009, pp. 45–48):

- The design and implementation of the program is innovative and seeks to build on traditional approaches to nursing education.
- The curriculum is flexible and reflects current societal and healthcare trends and issues, research findings, and innovative practices, as well as local and global perspectives.
- The curriculum is evidence based.
- The curriculum provides learning experiences that support evidence-based practice, multidisciplinary approaches to care, student achievement of clinical competence, and, as appropriate, expertise in specialty roles.
- The curriculum provides experiential cultural learning activities that enhance students' abilities to think critically, reflect

thoughtfully, and provide culturally sensitive, evidence-based nursing care to diverse populations.

■ The curriculum provides learning experiences that prepare graduates to assume roles that are essential to quality nursing practice, including but not limited to those of care provider, patient advocate, teacher, communicator, change agent, care coordinator, user of information technology, collaborator, and decision maker.

■ The innovativeness of the program helps create a preferred future for nursing.

■ Teaching/learning/evaluation strategies used by faculty are evidence based.

■ The educational environment empowers students and faculty and promotes collegial dialogue, innovation, change, creativity, values development, and ethical behavior.

Each of these ideas helps to provide an understanding of the functionality of the curriculum. It provides the framework from which the entire learning process should flow.

As faculty members consider the different aspects of curriculum, the types of learning (**Table 2-5**) should be contemplated. The six types of learning have been designated to provide a framework for leveling the learning that is planned within the curriculum. The initial three types of learning (**item**, **directive**, and **rational**) provide a "black-and-white" involvement with materials to be used. These three levels are considered to be at the technical levels of learning. The upper three types of learning (**syntactical**, **contextual**, and **inquiry**) strive to encourage critical thinking and a sense of investigation and analysis. As a curriculum is pulled together, faculty members should wisely consider what level of learning is appropriate at each stage within the learning process.

Once the levels of learning are determined, the curriculum can be fleshed out. Madeus and Stufflebeam (1989) provided four fundamental questions to be used when developing a curriculum:

1. What educational purposes should the school seek to attain?
2. What educational experiences can be provided that are likely to achieve these purposes?
3. How can these educational experiences be effectively organized?
4. How can we determine whether and to what extent these purposes are being attained?

The process of curriculum development must embrace several different levels within the educational process. The institution's **philosophy** of education provides the foundation for the entire educational

Table 2-5

Types of Learning

Type	Description
Item Learning	Focused on learning facts, pieces of information, individual aspects, straightforward associations; involuntary, automatic, and predictable
Directive Learning	Ascertaining of regulations, restrictions, and omissions; systems of directions that provide the "do's" and don'ts" for everyday jobs
Rational Learning	Introduces theory and the "why's" for doing things into the logical management of tasks; beginnings of the use of logic to influence judgment and decision making
Syntactical Learning	Investigation into the understanding of the whole; relationships and patterns are sought to guide unique client care; encourages individuals to make intuitive efforts as theory is meshed into practice
Contextual Learning	Inclusion of cultural aspects to frame the provision of care; symbols, political aspects, power, relationships, values, esthetic aspects, ethical perspectives, and philosophical facets are considered as transition into caring, compassionate, and positive care
Inquiry Learning	Resourcefulness, exploration, theorizing, strategizing, ascertaining, illuminating, and categorizing challenges and approaches to solve aspects of care; striving to find the foundations and questioning the process; demanding validation for aspects provided

Source: Adapted from Ironside, P. M. (Ed.). (2007). *On revolutions and revolutionaries: 25 years of reform and innovation in nursing education.* New York, NY: National League for Nursing.

experience at an institution. From this philosophy, the goals and aims within each designated program can be determined. Once the program has these aspects determined, specific instructional objectives and outcomes can be established that will provide the underpinning for task analysis, content selection, and learning activities.

Penn (2008) said it correctly when stating that "curriculum development is a dynamic process and requires continuous evaluation" (p. 160). The curriculum within schools of nursing is viewed as the responsibility of the faculty. The strengths and/or weaknesses of the learning plan are directly related to the effort put into the curriculum by each faculty member. It becomes imperative that faculty members understand and embrace the development and management of the curriculum within a school. According to Conway and Little (n.d.), "curriculum content should focus on what nurses do rather than where they work" (p. 3). Each member of the faculty has to appreciate and comprehend the nuances within the curriculum to effectively provide the guidance required within the learning environment. In light of the generational issues and the NLN's Hallmarks of Excellence, Speakman (2009) states "our programs and curricula must be student-centered, interactive, and innovative" (p. 44). To work within the boundaries of the learning environment, students must be empowered to learn. Instead of being thought of as pieces of clay or sponges within their seats, students need to be actively involved and central to the learning process. By embracing the idea of "colleagues in learning," each member becomes responsible for different components of the learning process. The responsibility for learning does not fall to one group of individuals. No longer can faculty members play the role of "sage on the stage"; they must be the "guides on the side." The curriculum must incorporate the idea that each participant (administration, faculty members, and students) in the learning environment has an active role in the learning process.

Committee Involvement

From the previous discussion about generational differences and curriculum, one can quickly see that characteristics of each generation will impact the role of faculty serving on **committees**. Whether faculty members are elected or appointed to committees, they still must be able to accomplish the **mission** and goals of the school. A simple solution to addressing differences would be to put all members of a generation into a single group. Unfortunately, this approach is nearly impossible and would also omit the rich diversity of opinions/perceptions necessary for embracing opportunities to grow and change in the fast-paced health arena. Thus, a mix of generations within faculty committees allows for creativity and innovation that is realistic and necessary for committee decisions and/or recommendations.

Recognizing the need for each generation's contribution to a committee, there are ways to utilize the generational characteristics so the committee can accomplish its goals. Since most committees have a chair to provide leadership, the chair can begin by identifying the generation to which each member belongs. Once the identification has been made, the work of the committee is considered (i.e., curriculum, student affairs, faculty affairs, admissions/progressions, etc.). The chair can then use Tables 2-1 and 2-3 to guide communication, feedback, and decisions for positive outcomes for the committee tasks. This allows for each generation of faculty members to participate and yet recognizes the differences inherent in each generation.

Tenure and Promotion

Achieving **tenure** and/or **promotion** is a quest for the majority of faculty members regardless of the type of educational institution. Perhaps at this point, tenure and promotion need to be discussed separately because not all faculty members will seek tenure. However, most faculty members at some point in time will pursue promotion.

Let's begin with the examination of tenure. It is important to keep in mind that, as mentioned, some faculty members do not wish to be on the tenure track. They choose to negotiate their faculty contract on a yearly basis. In addition, tenure is not easily obtained and all schools recognize the need for nontenured faculty. The nontenured faculty members should be recognized for their contributions.

Tenure is highly regarded and respected. It is considered to be both recognition and a reward for individual accomplishments over a designated period of time. Each school establishes the criteria for tenure. Obviously, each generation of faculty will have characteristics and work-related aspects (see Table 2-1 and 2-2) that will be of advantage to obtaining tenure.

Since tenure is based on specific criteria instituted by the school, the Veteran generation may achieve tenure easier than the other generations. The Veterans are disciplined, accept delayed rewards, and are hard working. Their values, strengths, and work ethics enhance their skills and abilities to obtain tenure.

The Baby Boomers are optimistic, driven, willing to take risks, and work efficiently. However, they believe time equals authority and they abhor conformity and rules. Since tenure is more than time in a position and requires specific criterion (rules), Baby Boomers may encounter difficulty achieving tenure.

The Gen Xers group is diverse, creative, self-starting, and output focused. This generation wants to get in, get the job done, and move on. Tenure requires patience and formal structure through specific criteria. Tenure would never be considered casual or fun.

Millennial individuals are realistic, competitive, outcome driven, and goal oriented. Their obsession with career development and desire to enhance work skills through continuing education are assets that assist them through the tenure process.

Promotion is one aspect of the role of the **academician** that most faculty members will pursue. There are two major reasons prompting faculty to seek promotion. Promotion can be viewed as a career ladder for faculty members that brings recognition to their work and accomplishments. Another reason to seek promotion is for financial gain. In most institutions, the only significant increase in salary is through promotion from one rank to the next. Thus, promotion is an honor and a reward for hard work. Again, Tables 2-1, 2-2, and 2-3 point out how each generation is successful in reaching the next highest rank. Veterans would view promotion more as an honor and a means for moving up in their career. The Baby Boomer lives to work, wants to "make a difference," and views career as a central focus. Gen Xers want a balanced life, work to live, and view careers as getting in the way of having fun. Millennials are optimistic, want to be evaluated on their work products, and perceive their careers to be always changing.

As a result of these generations' characteristics and work aspects, promotional efforts need to focus on the strengths of each. Promotion is possible for members of each generation but will require adherence to criteria established by individual schools. Again, this may cause stress for some but be motivating for others.

Policy and Procedure

A **policy** can be considered as a course of action—a plan. A **procedure** can be considered as the means to carry out the action/plan. Policies and procedures are a part of every aspect of the role of faculty in academia. The regents/trustees of the educational institution establish overall policies and procedures to govern the operation of the institution. In accordance with the institution, each school develops policies and procedures for faculty, staff, and students. Faculty members play an important role in the development, recommendations, and implementation of policies and procedures at the school and institutional levels. In the past, policies and procedures were based on "what's always been done." Currently, the emphasis is on evidence-based policies and procedures which allow for accurate, legal, and ethical considerations that are constantly changing with new information, new laws, and ethical situations that are emerging. Whether recommending, developing, or implementing policies, faculty members must be cognizant and diligent of the need for evidence to guide their decisions. The importance of that statement cannot be stressed enough. The nurse educator's role is grounded in policies and procedures on a daily basis, regardless of the setting—classroom, simulation lab, or student clinical experience.

Summary Thoughts

As we consider engaging the multigenerational groups currently found within the educational system, Hahns (2009) stated several tactics to generate a modification in constructing a healthy work environment: completing a self-assessment on a regular basis, pursuing knowledge about the generational differences, embracing the commonalities, and creating and establishing a culture of respect while endeavoring to bridge the generational gap that can exist. Another key aspect discussed in relation to generational differences is that of respect. Whereas the older generations establish respect based on years of experience and commitment to the activity, the younger generations place respect based upon engagement by the individuals and their ability and willingness to listen and mentor (Hahn, 2009; Tolbize, 2008; Wieck, 2008). Respect is earned by doing, not by number of years worked at a site. Conway and Little (n.d.) effectively articulate that faculty members must become facilitators, and students must increasingly develop a self-directed learner approach as education moves forward. No longer can students expect to be "spoon-fed" the necessary material. They must step up and take an active role. Faculty members must develop strategies to help the students to make this change in the educational environment.

In regard to curriculum, Speakman (2009) stated that "students will need to be engaged in student-centered curricula that are innovative and challenging, a curriculum both in the classroom and clinical setting that inspires a student to challenge assumptions, examine multiple methodologies of care and utilize current literature to frame their practice" (p. 46). Each faculty member must develop skills and commitment to embrace a student-centered curriculum which will challenge individuals to take an active part in the learning process. Students cannot be relegated to passively learning healthcare fundamentals at this time. Active involvement and commitment to learning on a continuous basis is paramount as health care moves forward.

To keep up with the momentum of change in health care, faculty members must provide valuable input on committees. Involvement gives faculty members a voice on important career-development aspects related to tenure and promotion as well as policies and procedures for governing the everyday work for nurse educators. Standards for policies and procedures must be evidence based. Research in nursing education must provide evidence to produce positive outcomes for students (see Chapter 10). Nursing faculty members are required to be knowledgeable of both clinical and educational research to keep up with the fast pace of health care and education in today's environment. The changes are related to the skills provided by students and the competencies required to practice nursing in a variety of settings.

Summary Points

1. For the first time in history, the workplace is engaged with four distinctive generational cohorts: Veterans, Baby Boomers, Generation Xers, and Millennials.

2. As with any grouping of individuals, the group members may display many of the same characteristics, but individuals will also have unique characteristics.

3. The Generation X and Millennial generations are considered to be technologically literate.

4. Faculty members should conscientiously consider the need to restructure course delivery to embrace the openness, civic focus, and self-reliant aspects presented by the Generation Xers and Millennial cohorts.

5. Faculty members must remember that the Millennial generation perceives education as being extremely expensive and thus must ensure that the majority of the educational process is viewed as realistic and meaningful.

6. Generation Xers look at the time to be committed to an experience, whereas the Millennials desire the uniqueness of the experience.

7. Both Generation Xers and Millennials expect to test authority repeatedly.

8. Generation Xers and Millennials seek to find individuals who have the experience and knowledge about how to get a message across.

9. The Millennial cohort treasures the ability to work with bright and energetic individuals.

10. Generation Xers appreciate freedom to approach problems and challenges in unique ways.

11. Communication and feedback are critical aspects of the learning process.

12. Generation Xers, overall, do not want public acknowledgement since they tend to be very private individuals.

13. Millennials want frequent feedback that is tied to goals and expectations.

14. As when working with any generation and culture, a sound knowledge of the group helps in understanding when and how group members can come to the table to work and/or learn.

15. Many different definitions can be found for the term curriculum.

16. Six types of learning have been identified: item, directive, rational, syntactical, contextual, and inquiry.

17. Once a program has determined the institutional philosophy, goals, and aims, specific instructional objectives and outcomes can be determined that will provide the underpinning for task analysis, content selection, and learning activities within a curriculum.

18. Curriculum development is a vigorous course of action and necessitates constant evaluation.

19. Within schools of nursing, curriculum is viewed as the responsibility of the faculty cohort.

20. The responsibility for learning does not fall to one group of individuals.

21. Each faculty member must develop skills and commitment to embrace a student-centered curriculum that will challenge individuals to take an active part in the learning process.
22. Faculty members from each generation provide a rich diversity necessary to achieve committee work.
23. The committee leadership (chair) must draw on the characteristics of each faculty generation to fulfill the committee tasks.
24. Tenure is the achievement of school-determined criteria for a designated period of time and is highly regarded and respected.
25. Not all faculty members will pursue tenure.
26. Promotion brings recognition and financial gains for faculty members.
27. Policies and procedures are a daily occurrence for nurse educators and must be based on solid evidence.

Tips for Nurse Educators to Use

1. Faculty members are dealing with the challenge of embracing and respecting the different generational needs within the faculty and student cohorts.
2. Faculty members must develop a sound foundational knowledge about generational strengths and challenges to ensure the success of the educational process while decreasing the frustrations that emerge when conflict and stress are present.
3. Faculty members must conscientiously consider the need to restructure course delivery to embrace the openness, civic focus, and self-reliant aspects within the Generation X and Millennial groups.
4. Material presented must be practical and realistic.
5. Clear delineation as to the rationale for each experience needs to be addressed, thus providing value for the encounter.
6. Generation Xers expect freedom to investigate innovative ways to address challenges and/or problems.
7. Generation Xers do not like teams and groups because singularity is a main principle in their value system.
8. Millennials desire teams and groups to be used to address the challenges presented in the classroom and clinical sites.
9. Email and voicemail are the primary means for communication used by the Generation X and Millennial groups.
10. Messages should be directed toward outcomes and goals/aspirations to gain support for the management of the interaction.
11. The Millennial generation strives to learn by questioning.
12. Faculty members would benefit by having a time at the beginning of courses for clarifying and validating the goals and expectations.

13. Developing generationally sensitive styles to effectively coach and motivate all members of the healthcare team is desired.
14. Active listing is imperative.
15. The learning types of item, directive, and rational are seen as fact-oriented learning.
16. The learning types of syntactical, contextual, and inquiry encourage critical thinking and a sense of investigation and analysis.
17. Each member of the faculty has to appreciate and comprehend the nuances within the curriculum to effectively provide the guidance required within the learning environment.
18. Students need to be actively involved and central to the learning process.
19. Utilize the strengths of your generational characteristics to plan your career development for tenure and/or promotion.
20. Become familiar with the policies and procedures of your educational institution, school, and clinical facilities where your students are assigned.
21. Provide feedback by taking an active role on committees at all levels of your institution, using the unique perspectives from your generational cohort.

References

Conway, J., & Little, P. (n.d.). From practice to theory: Reconceptualising curriculum development for PBL. Australia: University of Newcastle.

Hahn, J. (2009). Effectively manage a multigenerational staff. Nursing Management, 8–10.

Hammill, G. (2005). Mixing and managing four generations of employees. FDUMagazine Online. Retrieved November 24, 2009, from www.fdu.edu/newspubs/magazine/05ws/generations.htm

Ironside, P. M. (Ed.). (2007). On revolutions and revolutionaries: 25 years of reform and innovation in nursing education. New York, NY; National League for Nursing.

Madeus, G. F., & Stufflebeam, D. L. (1989). Educational evaluation: The work of Ralph Tyler. Boston, MA: Kluwer Academic Press.

O'Connor, M. (2009).Social networking and the role of technology in nursing education. Voice of Nursing Leadership, 7(6), 8–9.

Oliva, P. F. (1988). Developing the curriculum (2nd ed.). Glenview, IL: Scott, Foresman and Company.

Penn, B. K. (2008). Mastering the teaching role: A guide for nurse educators. Philadelphia, PA: F.A. Davis Company.

Sherman, R. O. (2006). Leading a multigenerational nursing workforce: Issues, challenges, and strategies. OJIN: The Online Journal of Issues in Nursing, 11(2). Manuscript 2. Available online at www.nursingworld.org/MainMenuCategories/ANAMarketplace/ANAPeriodicals/OJIN/TableofContents/Volum112006/No2May06/tpc30_216074.aspx

Speakman, E. (2009). Student-centered, interactive, innovative programs and curricula: Needed to achieve excellence in nursing education. In M. H. Adams & R. M. Valiga (Eds.), Achieving excellence in nursing education (Chapter 5). New York, NY: National League for Nursing.

Tolbize, A. (2008). Generational differences in the workplace. In Research and Training Center on Community Living. University of Minnesota.

Wieck, K. L. (2008). Managing the millennials. Nurse Leader, 6(6), 26–29.

Wieck, K. L., Dols, J., & Northam, S. (2009). What nurses want: The nurse incentives project. Nurse Economic$, 27(3), 169–177, 201.

Web Links

The National League for Nursing's Hallmark of Excellence is available at www.nln.org/excellence/hallmarks_indicators.htm.

The National League for Nursing's Excellence in Nursing Education Model is available at www.nln.org/excellence/model/index.htm.

Multiple Choice Questions

1. The four generation cohorts currently present in the workplace are
   A. Veterans, Baby Boomers, Generation S, Millennials.
   B. Veterans, Baby Busters, Generation X, Millennials.
   C. Victorian, Baby Boomers, Generation X, Millennials.
   D. Veterans, Baby Boomers, Generation X, Millennials.

   Rationale:

   The four cohorts currently present in the workplace are the Veterans, the Baby Boomers, Generation X, and Millennials (Hahn, 2009; Wieck, 2008).

2. The different generations can have an influence on
   A. development of teams.
   B. discouragement.
   C. decreasing efficiency.
   D. management of stress.

   Rationale:

   Hammill (2005) states that generational dissimilarities can influence everything from recruiting and fostering teams to managing change and encouraging, overseeing, and developing efficiency and output.

3. In regard to managing issues, the Baby Boomers tend to rely on
   A. an open-slate approach.
   B. group activities.
   C. tested ways.
   D. mentors.

   Rationale:

   The tested ways are embraced by the Baby Boomers, whereas an open slate for managing the issues is celebrated by the Generation X group. Baby Boomer faculty members must allow the Gen X group to try out new approaches while respecting the teamwork orientation found within the Millennials.

4. Generation X individuals tend to prefer
   A. individual work.
   B. group work.
   C. a mixture of both individual and group work.
   D. neither individual nor group work.

   Rationale:

   Gen X individuals do not like teams and groups since singularity is a main principle in their value system. According to Wieck (2008), "the team orientation of the Millennials is in stark contrast to the more independent-minded Gen X" (p. 27). Millennial individuals desire teams and groups to be used to address the challenges presented in the classroom and clinical sites.

5. The Millennial cohort tends to communicate

  A. with diplomacy and directness.
  B. with politeness and active involvement.
  C. with bluntness and directness.
  D. in a discrete and logical manner.

Rationale:

The Baby Boomers communicate with diplomacy and directness. Millennials desire communication that is polite and active in nature. Generation Xers, on the other hand, did not develop as many of the networking skills, thus they expect blunt, immediate messages. See Table 2-4.

6. Generation Xers want messages to be tied to

  A. goals and aspirations.
  B. consensus statements.
  C. outcomes.
  D. interactions.

Rationale:

Another interesting communication aspect is that Gen Xers want the messages tied to the outcomes, whereas Millennials value messages that are connected to goals and aspirations. This focus for the messages could be very valuable as faculty members strive to communicate with the different members within a class. Messages should be directed toward outcomes and goals/aspirations to gain support for the management of the interaction. See Table 2-4.

7. Feedback for Millennials should be

  A. tied to goals and provided often.
  B. tied to freedom from public recognition.
  C. public in nature.
  D. subtle and private in nature.

Rationale:

Generation Xers overall do not want public acknowledgement since they tend to be very private individuals. Feedback to this group should be regular, constructive, and allow for freedom. Millennials want frequent feedback that is tied to their focus on goals and expectations. Communication, feedback, and interactions should concentrate on management and attainment of the goals and expectations established. See Table 2-4.

8. Curricula are viewed as

A. conceptual frameworks that are not useful in everyday life.
B. documents that reflect the students' values and aims.
C. written documents used to direct the learning process.
D. written documents used to direct the accreditation process.

Rationale:

Each of these definitions implies written documents that are used to direct the learning process. Ironside (2007) takes a slightly different approach to the idea: "The most common agreement seems to be that curriculum is what actually occurs between and among persons in the educational enterprise and not some 'plan' for learning that is reflected in written materials" (p. 78). Curriculum moves from a document into a working process whereby learning can occur.

9. The learning types of item, directive, and rational serve to provide support for:

A. technical levels of learning.
B. the development of critical thinking.
C. all types of learning.
D. everyday learning.

Rationale:

The initial three types of learning (item, directive, and rational) provide a "black-and-white" involvement with materials to be used. These three levels are considered to be at the technical level of learning. See Table 2-5.

10. Committees composed of members of each generation provide

A. dissention and chaos.
B. diversity and realism.
C. an environment of disagreement.
D. unrealistic decisions.

Rationale:

A mix of the generations for faculty membership on committees allows for creativity and innovation that is realistic and necessary for committee decisions and/or recommendations.

11. Tenure is a process that

A. occurs only in university settings.
B. all faculty members seek.
C. can only be obtained by the Veteran generation.
D. is based on specific criteria.

Rationale:

Tenure occurs in all educational settings but is not sought by every faculty member. Some generations have characteristics that enhance their ability to achieve the specific criteria established by each school.

12. Promotion provides faculty members a method to:

    A. gain recognition and a significant increase in salary.
    B. give only one generation an opportunity to move up a career ladder.
    C. improve their community image.
    D. plan to decrease their stress.

Rationale:

Promotion can be viewed as a career ladder used to gain recognition and a higher salary. Promotion is possible for all generations but will require strict adherence to criteria established by individual schools, which may cause stress for some faculty members but motivation for others.

13. Policies and procedures are

    A. a necessary nuisance in all settings.
    B. a method to control faculty input.
    C. a part of every aspect of the role of faculty members in academia.
    D. based on "what's always been done" and do not require evidence.

Rationale:

Policies and procedures are a part of every aspect of the role of faculty in academia. Faculty members play an important role in the development, recommendation, and implementation of policies and procedures that must be evidence based.

14. Evidence required for policies and procedures must

    A. be necessary in only the clinical settings.
    B. not be influenced by changes in the healthcare arena.
    C. include accurate legal and ethical considerations.
    D. address only matters that concern students' competence.

Rationale:

Currently, the emphasis is on evidence-based policies and procedures that allow for accurate legal and ethical considerations that are constantly changing with new information, new laws, and ethical situations.

15. Knowledge of faculty regarding clinical and educational research is

    A. only required for faculty members involved in research.

    B. too much for faculty members to handle in today's fast-paced environment.

    C. nice to have but not necessary in the classroom, only in the clinical setting.

    D. **a requirement to provide students with the competencies to practice nursing in a variety of settings**.

Rationale:

All nursing faculty members are required to be cognizant of both clinical and educational research to keep up with the fast pace of health care and education in today's environment while still providing students with the competencies needed to practice nursing in a variety of settings.

Discussion Questions

1. From the materials provided within the chapter and tables, select at least five to six characteristics that you think must be included in a plan to effectively address the needs and expectations for the different generational groups within a classroom experience.

Considerations:

In Tables 2-1, 2-2, 2-3, and 2-4, select several characteristics from each of the columns to help determine a plan for meeting the educational needs related to the different generational groups.

2. From the materials provided within the chapter and tables, select at least five to six characteristics that you think must be included in a plan to effectively address the needs and expectations for the different generational groups within a clinical setting experience.

Considerations:

In Tables 2-1, 2-2, 2-3, and 2-4, select several characteristics from each of the columns to help determine a plan for meeting the educational needs related to the different generational groups.

3. From the materials provided within the chapter and tables, select at least five to six characteristics that you think must be included in a plan to effectively address the needs and expectations for the different generational groups within a faculty committee.

Considerations

See Tables 2-1 and 2-2, and develop a plan that you as a chairperson would use to get all of the generational members to participate on the committee in a positive, functional manner.

4. Obtain examples of institutional policies and procedures for tenure and/or promotion. Establish criteria for your school that consider these policies and procedures while providing opportunities for growth of nursing faculty members.

Considerations:

Carefully consider the current policies and procedures in place within institutions of higher learning. Investigate which statements within the documents are based upon evidence. Consider what level of evidence would be appropriate for this type of document.

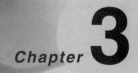

Chapter **3**

The Teaching Experience in Nursing

Theresa M. "Terry" Valiga

Chapter Objectives

At the conclusion of this chapter, the learner will be able to:

1. Describe the major tenets of at least three learning theories.
2. Explain how knowledge of the concept of *learning style* can enhance teacher effectiveness.
3. Trace the evolution of the role of teacher from provider of information/facts (i.e., "sage on the stage") to facilitator of learning (i.e., "guide on the side")
4. Articulate one's own philosophy of or approach to teaching with reflection of values associated with the philosophy.
5. Propose strategies to develop one's knowledge and skills related to implementation of the nurse educator role.

Key Terms

➤ Adult learning principles

➤ Andragogy

➤ Brain-based learning

➤ Collaborative and cooperative learning

➤ Educator

➤ Learning style   ➤ Teacher

➤ Pedagogy

Introduction

As noted in Chapter 2, educators practice in colleges and universities and are expected to be "good citizens of the academy." Such "good citizenship" requires that educators be effective teachers and advisors. They also are responsible for participating in and contributing to the work of committees at the discipline (i.e., nursing) level and at the broader (i.e., department/college or university) level. Educators also are expected to design, implement, and evaluate the curricula in their discipline, taking into account the institution's mission, goals, and degree requirements. In addition, they are responsible for developing, implementing, evaluating, and revising (as needed) policies and procedures related to a number of areas, such as student admission, progression, and graduation; peer review; and tenure and promotion.

Indeed, the responsibilities of an academician are complex and broad. More important, they are ever-evolving. This chapter provides an overview of how the role of the academic educator has changed over time, some of the issues that currently face faculty, and the uniqueness of the nurse educator role. It is intended to provide a broad context for discussions that follow—discussions related to classroom, online, and clinical teaching; program evaluation; competency assessment; and future directions for nursing education. Finally, it is intended to challenge the reader to "do philosophy" (Greene, 1973) and reflect on her or his values as a teacher and educator.

Historical Background

There have always been **teachers** in our world. Parents teach their children values, skills, and ways of interacting with others. Religious leaders teach us about religious practices and beliefs. Community leaders teach us how we can contribute to the health and viability of our communities. And "school marms" teach students about the world in which they live.

Educators, however, are something else. They are the individuals whose professional responsibility and major contribution to society relate to enhancing the total development of learners—their minds, their values, their skills—and to advancing knowledge and understanding in their field. These are individuals who have prepared for the role, who engage in a continual study of how to be most effective in that role, and who provide leadership within the educational community.

From the days of Socrates, educators have lived among us. Socrates, for example, spent his time talking with the youth of ancient Greek society using methods that stimulated them to think in new ways, to consider new possibilities, to contemplate deep issues, and to ponder the future and how they might influence it. There were no structured classrooms, there were no course syllabi, there were no rank or tenure systems, and there were few books from which to seek facts. Instead, knowledge and understanding were gained from deep thinking, and the role of the educator was to stimulate, guide, and challenge such thinking.

As societies evolved and there came to be a growing recognition of the need to educate more individuals who could lead those societies, educational systems began to be more structured. Tutors were employed to teach the children of aristocrats, and "public" schools were created to teach the children of less noble families. The responsibilities of such tutors or public school teachers were to help students learn to read, write, calculate, and understand the history of their world, which was being documented more carefully through textbooks, research reports, and presentations by experts. In some instances, individuals were prepared—often in an apprentice-type system, where they learned "at the elbow" of a master in the craft—for a specific role, such as physician, lawyer, or clergyman.

The focus of education was on the youth of society, assuming, perhaps, that adults were established in life and had no desire or need to learn. Because the number of children continued to grow, more efficient systems of education needed to be created. There seemed to be an assumption that all children needed to learn the same thing and in the same way, and that all should progress through this newly formed educational system in the same way and at the same pace. No attention was paid to individualized learning, self-paced learning, or mastery learning; and those who could not "keep up" because of physical or mental disability, lack of commitment or interest, lack of aptitude to do the work, or inability or unwillingness to "follow the rules" of the system were "let go."

Those involved in such practices who were true educators, however, began to question the systems that were in place. They reflected on the nature of learning, the conditions that encouraged or got in the way of learning, and the role of the teacher. Theories of learning began to emerge, the role of the teacher/educator began to be more carefully defined, and the larger purposes of schooling began to be articulated.

Learning Theories and Approaches

Theories of learning can be categorized, generally, into several areas—behavioral, cognitive, humanistic, and brain-based. Each of these will be explained briefly, and the ways in which our thinking about learning have evolved will be noted.

Behavioral theories of learning, espoused by scientists such as Skinner (1974), explained that learning was little more than a response to a stimulus. Learning was thought to be a form of operant conditioning (as articulated by Pavlov), and the role of the teacher was to manipulate the environment and be a "reinforcement machine" by providing rewards for "good" behavior or punishment for "bad" behavior. The basic premise was that a behavior would continue or be extinguished, depending on what was rewarded or punished.

In contrast to this perspective that placed emphasis on external factors, cognitive learning theories posited that learning had to do with what went on inside the learner's head. They argued that rewards and punishment were not necessary to facilitate learning, but what would stimulate learning was an environment that presented the learner with disequilibrium, imbalance, and tension. Indeed, scientists such as Gagne (1965) noted that past experiences, perceptions, and ways of incorporating and thinking about information created tension in the learner and affected learning.

Many of us are familiar with the work of Piaget (Atherton, 2009), who focused on cognitive processes and rational approaches to solving problems and how those processes and approaches evolved. Piaget studied children and outlined four stages of cognitive development, the highest of which was achieved by the mid-teen years. He noted that a child acquires knowledge by interacting with his or her physical and psychological environment.

The work of Piaget was challenged, in part, by Perry (1970), who asserted that cognitive/intellectual development is not achieved by the mid-teen years but continues into adulthood and, in fact, happens over and over again when individuals are placed in new situations that require knowledge and understanding they do not possess. Perry outlined a nine-stage model in which an individual moves from a dualistic, right/wrong perspective—where the world and problems in it are thought to have a single right answer known to some authority figure—to a more relativistic perspective, where one can appreciate and accept that different situations or circumstances lead one to hold views and make decisions that may be more varied, realizing that there may be more than one "right answer." One moves along this continuum, Perry said, by being challenged with thinking that is one stage higher than one's current position, while being supported through the cognitive struggles such challenges create.

Perhaps one of the best-known authorities on learning was John Dewey (1916), who proposed that knowledge is acquired through discovery and experimentation. He asserted that if given enough time and guidance, almost anyone could learn anything. According to Dewey, then, the goal of education and educators was/is to actively involve learners in discovering processes and relationships, and giving them enough time and "freedom" to experiment, make mistakes, reflect on those mistakes, and eventually understand and comprehend the material under investigation.

The idea of active involvement and discovery was expanded by educational theorists such as Bandura (1977), who proposed that individuals learn from observing others and paying attention to what happens to them. Role modeling is important in social learning theory, and there is acknowledgement that individuals other than the assigned teacher could be the role model and the source of learning. The environment for learning and all those in that environment were now identified as significant to learning.

Learning with and through others, as noted by Bandura, is congruent with the need to be more humanistic, rather than behavioristic, in our approaches to teaching and learning. As noted by Carl Rogers (1969), teachers need to attend to learners' feelings, draw on their life experiences, and strive to help them grow personally and be fulfilled as individuals. With this perspective in mind, educators construct learning environments in which the learner participates completely and has control over what, how, when, and even where he or she learns. In essence, the educator transitions from being a "sage on the stage" to a "guide on the side," trusting the learner to confront problems in thoughtful ways, being open to changing his or her way of thinking, and engaging in critical self-evaluation. In essence, the learning process is thought to be more significant than the specifics of what is learned.

A focus on the learning process is evident in current research that focuses on ways in which our brains work and how that influences how we learn, the environments that enhance our learning, the extent to which we retain or lose bits of information, and the ways in which we are able to make connections among what we know. Such **brain-based learning** theories (Jensen, 2008) build on the notions posited in the 1970s regarding left- and right-brain thinking:

> Left-brain thinking was described as analytic, logical, linear, and rule-bound. It calls upon mathematical and verbal skills,

focuses on parts more so than wholes, and allows us to dis-
criminate and be explicit. This is the paradigm that has domi-
nated our culture in general and our educational systems in
particular.

Right-brain thinking was described as artistic, holistic, and
integrative. It involves feelings, intuition and insight, and does
not necessarily require verbal or math skills. The right brain
allows us to integrate ideas into wholes, which are seen as
more important than individual parts, and to look for tacit
understanding of situations. This paradigm is culturally sup-
pressed and not particularly evident in out educational systems.

Later, scientists proposed that the brain evolved in three parts: the
lower brain, where survival learning occurs; the mid-brain, where
emotions reside; and the upper brain, where higher-order thinking
takes place. Current brain-based education embraces a more holistic
view of the brain—one that is more systems-based and *gestalt* in
nature—where the whole is greater than the sum of its parts.

Neuroscientists have done autopsies, experiments, and various
types of scans (e.g., MRIs) to conduct research that has implications
for improved teaching practices. We are coming to better understand
how human learning actually occurs, how the brain processes and
retains information. At present, this research has led to the identification of the following core principles to guide brain-based education
(Jensen, 2008):

- The brain is a parallel processor that can perform several activi-
  ties at once.
- The brain perceives wholes and parts simultaneously.
- Information is stored in multiple areas of the brain and can
  be retrieved through multiple memory and neural pathways.
- Learning engages the whole body; thus, all learning is mind–
  body in nature.
- Humans' search for meaning is innate.
- The search for meaning comes through patterning.
- Emotions are critical to patterning, and they drive our atten-
  tion, meaning, and memory.
- Meaning is more important than just information.
- Learning involves focused attention and peripheral
  perception.
- We have two types of memory: spatial and rote.
- We understand best when facts are embedded in natural spatial
  memory.
- The brain is social and develops better in concert with other
  brains.

- Complex learning is enhanced by challenge and inhibited by stress.
- Every brain in uniquely organized.
- Learning is developmental.

A review of this list of core principles would seem to suggest that the theorists discussed earlier were all correct—to some extent. Meaning is important. We learn through focused attention as well as through exploration. Education must attend to the whole student, where learning with others is effective and each learner is unique. Indeed, findings from brain-based research and educational literature in general now embrace much of the work of the pioneers in educational theory.

Today, we hear calls for **collaborative and cooperative learning**. We are tasked with providing learners with problems that challenge them to construct new ideas or concepts—based on what they know and what they seek to find out—that allow them to manage those problems. And, among other things, we hear calls for more humanism in education, where learners' feelings and experiences are valued as important and acknowledged to lead to personal growth. The role of the educator who is guided by such perspectives, therefore, is to facilitate learning, rather than be the all-knowing authority who conveys information. So how do we do that as nurse educators?

Current Educational Practices and Challenges

Humanistic learning perspectives (Rogers, 1969) and brain-based learning theorists (Jensen, 2008) have led educators to see their central purpose as fostering curiosity, enthusiasm, initiative, and responsibility for one's own learning, rather than forcing the mastery of isolated facts. Knowles (1978), the "father" of adult learning, expanded these basic principles to identify characteristics of adult learners that must be attended to if learning is to be successful. Among those **adult learning principles** are the following:

- Allow adult learners to exercise autonomy and self-direction in the learning process.
- Help adult learners achieve the personal learning goals they have identified.
- Ensure that all learning experiences designed for adults are relevant.
- Encourage adult learners to solve practical problems.
- Develop learning experiences that build on the life experiences of adult learners.
- Help adult learners fulfill their potential.

As a result of his work with adult learners, Knowles introduced the concept of **andragogy**, which he defined as the education of adults. He asserted that the andragogical approach is learner-directed, focused on "the tasks of life," immediately applicable, and focused on learning how to learn. This, he proposed, is in direct contrast with the concept of **pedagogy**, which he defined as the education of children. A pedagogical approach calls for the learner to be passive, the subject matter to be central, motivation to come from external rewards, and learning to be focused on the future (i.e., "You'll need to know this someday").

In recent years, the line between andragogy and pedagogy has become blurred, and the term *pedagogy* is now receiving increased attention and being used widely. Educators are realizing that the principles initially outlined for adult learners have significance for any learner, regardless of age. Additionally, the term *pedagogy* has come to refer more to the art and science of teaching than it does to the learners engaged in the teaching/learning process (i.e., children or adults). We also hear talk of *critical pedagogy*, which focuses on helping learners question and challenge the dominant ways of thinking in our society— the beliefs and practices that dominate, and the "sacred cows" that are embedded in our educational systems. We acknowledge publicly that learning is not an automatic consequence of teaching, but results from sound pedagogy that has been deliberately designed to promote learning. Indeed, part of that deliberate design is to base one's educational approaches on research findings, thereby engaging in evidence-based teaching practices.

Today's students are increasingly diverse regarding culture, ethnic backgrounds, language abilities, and past educational experiences. They are technologically savvy and want to be fully engaged with and see relevance in the material under study. In other words, they want all learning experiences to have meaning for them. Additionally, the students of today have a wide variety of learning styles.

Learning Styles

Learning styles can be thought of as the unique ways in which individuals perceive, interact with, process, and respond to information and learning situations. They involve cognitive, affective, and physiological factors. Learning styles are thought to be relatively stable over time. All individuals learn through all modalities, but each of us prefers one or several over the others.

Gardner (1999) labeled these approaches to learning as "intelligences." He originally outlined seven such intelligences:

■ Verbal/Linguistic: Individuals with this preference prefer to read, write, talk, and share, and they "think in words."

■ Mathematical/Logical: These learners prefer to work with numbers, solve problems, experiment, ask questions, and think "logically" about solutions to problems or answers to questions.

■ Visual/Spatial: Learners who have strength in this area of intelligence "think in pictures." They prefer to draw, view pictures, create designs or models, think through mazes, and read.

■ Bodily-Kinesthetic: Individuals who have strength here prefer to move around, feel or manipulate things, use tools, dance, and use many senses.

■ Musical: Learners who have strength in this area of intelligence "think in rhythms," preferring to pick out patterns, make up songs to help them remember, and listen to music.

■ Interpersonal: These learners have many friends and like to talk to people, join and work in groups, share material and knowledge, collaborate with others, and resolve conflicts.

■ Intrapersonal: Individuals who have strength in this area of intelligence prefer to work alone. They think deeply, are reflective, are comfortable with independent or self-paced activities, are aware of their own values, recognize their own strengths and weaknesses, and work diligently to pursue their personal interests and goals.

Recently, Gardner also noted that some learners are naturalistic (i.e., preferring to engage with nature to enhance learning) and some are existential (i.e., learning best from explorations of the lived experiences of human beings).

Many others have described learning styles. Gregorc (1984) described four types of learners:

■ concrete/sequentials, who prefer structure and quiet environments;

■ abstract/sequentials, who are global thinkers and need many facts;

■ abstract/random learners, who anchor their thinking processes in feelings and ask questions randomly, preferring a busy environment; and

■ concrete/random learners, who are inquisitive, make intuitive leaps, and are more concerned with "why" than with "how."

Perhaps the most widely used framework is that outlined by Kolb (1984). He identified the following types of learning styles:

■ convergent, where the learner prefers problem solving and practical application—the thinkers and doers;

■ divergent, where the learner prefers to organize specific relationships into a meaningful whole and generate alternative ideas—the feelers and watchers;

■ assimilative, where the learner prefers to reason, create models, and "play" with ideas—the watchers and thinkers; and

■ accommodative, where the learner prefers to do things, take risks, and rely on others for specific information—the doers and feelers.

Kolb noted that learning is a continuous process that is grounded in experience and is, by its very nature, full of tension.

Despite all of this work related to defining and measuring learning styles, questions and misconceptions remain. First of all, research does not support many of the claims and assumptions underlying learning style constructs. Second, attempting to match teaching strategies with specific learning styles is very difficult and does not often result in improved learning. Third, most learners are multimodal and learn in a variety of ways. Finally, as education moves toward more cooperative and collaborative learning environments, it may be more important to think about group dynamics and group interaction than the learning styles of individuals within those groups.

As educators, it may be valuable to help learners identify their own preferences for learning so that they can use that information most effectively. However, both we and they must be careful not to "pigeon-hole" individuals into a single style and fail to challenge learners through a variety of experiences. We must realize that we, too, have our own preferences for how we learn. Those preferences influence how we teach. Therefore, it is essential that educators be attuned to designing learning experiences and evaluation methods that "tap into" many senses, are varied and do not advantage or disadvantage any particular group of students, and reflect the insights gained from pedagogical research efforts.

One thing that does evolve from all of these theories and all of the research on learning is a set of guiding principles that was formulated more than 20 years ago, but still has relevance today. In 1987—in response to criticisms of higher education (i.e., apathetic students, illiterate graduates, incompetent teaching, impersonal campuses)—Chickering and Gamson led a group of educators on a journey to define how students and faculty members could improve undergraduate education. They reviewed 50 years of research on "the way teachers teach and students learn, how students work and play with one another, and how students and faculty talk to each other" (Chickering & Gamson, 1987, p. 1).

The result of this careful and thorough analysis was the formulation of seven principles for good practice in undergraduate education. Though the focus of this work was on the undergraduate experience, the principles also apply to graduate education. In addition, the principles have been supported through research that has been done since their publication, which attests to their timelessness and significance. Those seven principles for good practice in education are as follows:

- Encourage student–faculty contact: Interaction between teachers and students is the most important factor in engaging students with the material to be studied and facilitating their learning.
- Encourage cooperation among students: Learning is enhanced when it feels like a team effort rather than a solo race. Good learning is collaborative and social, not competitive and isolated.
- Encourage active learning: Learning is not a spectator sport! Students must make what they learn part of themselves, and they do so by being actively engaged.
- Give prompt feedback: Knowing what you know and do not know focuses learning. Learning is dependent on frequent feedback if it is to be sustained, practice if it is to be nourished, and opportunities to use what has been learned if it is to have meaning.
- Emphasize time on task: Learning to use one's time well is critical to effective learning, and students may need help in learning effective time management skills.
- Communicate high expectations: Expecting students to perform well becomes a self-fulfilling prophecy, so teachers must "set the bar high" and then work with students to help them achieve that goal.
- Respect students' diverse talents and ways of learning: Students bring different talents and styles of learning to the learning experience. They need opportunities to show their talents and their intelligences (Gardner, 1999), and to learn in ways that work best for them.

The individual who routinely and thoughtfully employs these principles of good education in combination with insights gained from a study of various learning theories is well positioned to evolve as an effective educator.

Competencies of Nurse Educators

In essence, educators need to strive to create learning systems that are learner-centered, focus on inquiry, attend to the total development of the learner, actively involve learners, call upon many senses, and challenge learners to think about their thinking. Learning together, educators and learners need to allow for individualized learning, encourage expression and exploration of personal feelings and values, provide opportunities to work and learn in teams, and constantly raise questions about the world around us.

The role of the educator is to facilitate learning, encourage collaboration, help students learn how to learn, empower learners, challenge students to take responsibility for their own learning, and encourage and support a spirit of inquiry. Of course, the educator also gives information, helps learners know where and how to find information on their own, and helps them develop skills to critique and judge the information they find. Educators assess learning needs, create positive and empowering learning environments, provide feedback, coach, inspire, challenge, and genuinely care about the learners and their success. The role we assume as educators is influenced in large part by our philosophy; thus, it is important for educators to "do philosophy" so that we can be most effective in the role.

What does it mean to "do philosophy," and why is it important? Greene (1973), an educational philosopher, challenged educators to "do philosophy" by taking the risk of thinking about what we do when we teach, and what we mean when we talk of enabling others to learn. She also challenged educators to look, if we can, at our presuppositions and to examine critically the principles underlying what we think and what we say as educators. Although Green laid out these challenges more than 35 years ago, they are still relevant today. In fact, they have been presented over and again—though with different words or changing emphases—by educational scholars, including Palmer (2007).

In his personal account of his journey as a teacher, Palmer (2007) concluded that "good teachers must live examined lives and try to understand what animates their actions for better and for worse" (p. ix). He talked about the importance of knowing those whom we teach and being connected to them, knowing ourselves because "we teach who we are" (p. xi), and trusting ourselves and all those engaged in the educational enterprise. Palmer's basic premise is that "good teaching cannot be reduced to technique; good teaching comes from the identity and integrity of the teacher" (p. 10). Thus, one's personal philosophy and self-understanding are critical to effective teaching.

Although we often have to ask and answer painful questions to "do philosophy," we must think about what we are doing in order to be most effective at what we are doing. Do we not ask our students to reflect on their values, what drives them, and how the assumptions they make about themselves and others affect the care they provide? We can do no less. Such a "heightened self-consciousness and greater clarity" (Greene, 1973, p. 11) about our philosophy of education and our conceptualizations about teaching and learning will enhance the teaching experience in nursing and help us successfully achieve and continually improve our competence in the role.

The educator competencies we need to develop and continually refine were articulated by the National League for Nursing (2005) and further explicated by Halstead (2007). They include the following:

- Facilitate Learning: Nurse educators are responsible for creating an environment in classroom, laboratory, and clinical settings that facilitates student learning and the achievement of desired cognitive, affective, and psychomotor outcomes.
- Facilitate Learner Development and Socialization: Nurse educators recognize their responsibility for helping students develop as nurses and integrate the values and behaviors expected of those who fulfill that role.
- Use Assessment and Evaluation Strategies: Nurse educators use a variety of strategies to assess and evaluate student learning in classroom, laboratory, and clinical settings, as well as in all domains of learning.
- Participate in Curriculum Design and Evaluation of Program Outcomes: Nurse educators are responsible for formulating program outcomes and designing curricula that reflect contemporary healthcare trends and prepare graduates to function effectively in the healthcare environment.
- Function as a Change Agent and Leader: Nurse educators function as change agents and leaders to create a preferred future for nursing education and nursing practice.
- Pursue Continuous Quality Improvement in the Nurse Educator Role: Nurse educators recognize that their role is multidimensional and that an ongoing commitment to develop and maintain competence in the role is essential.
- Engage in Scholarship: Nurse educators acknowledge that scholarship is an integral component of the faculty role, and that teaching itself is a scholarly activity.
- Function Within the Educational Environment: Nurse educators are knowledgeable about the educational environment

within which they practice and recognize how political, institutional, social, and economic forces impact their role.

As educators, we must have a sound knowledge base about teaching and learning so that we can most effectively help our increasingly diverse students learn the complexities of what it means to be a nurse and to engage in the practice of nursing. We must continually refine our teaching skills so that we can develop effective case studies, games, simulations, discussions, online resources, lectures, visuals, group projects, values clarification exercises, and clinical learning experiences.

Such ongoing development and improvement as educators will occur through deliberate efforts. Just as clinicians continually keep current and advance their knowledge and skills related to practice and the care of the patients for whom they provide care, so, too, must educators keep current and advance their knowledge and skills related to the practice of teaching and the ways they interact with and guide the total development of their students. How can such ongoing development occur?

One route to continued growth as an educator is to enroll in academic courses that are relevant. Courses in innovative teaching practices, the integration of technology into nursing education, building the science of nursing education, new advances in clinical education, the history and current issues facing higher education, or other relevant topics are all areas that need to be considered.

Additionally, there are many professional conferences offered for educators. Examples of educational activities that can be used to support and prepare the educator are: conferences and webinars offered by the National League for Nursing (NLN) and the American Association of Colleges of Nursing (AACN), as well as those offered by the Association for Research in Higher Education, American Association of Higher Education, other national organizations, and individual colleges/universities. At such conferences, educators are introduced to the latest innovative practices and research efforts. They have opportunities to engage in dialogue with others in that same role.

The number of books about education, teaching strategies, evaluation of learning, brain-based research, and so on is ever-increasing. Nurse educators would do well to engage with this literature outside our own field. In medicine, for example, there is a fair amount of research being done about new curriculum designs, the use of simulation, and collaborative learning. In addition, we can learn a great deal from educators in business who have extensive experience with problem-focused education, where students work in groups to complete projects that have real-world relevance and use. And literature related to broad education goals—such as those often associated with the arts and humanities—keep educators "grounded" in the fact that our purpose is more than to prepare students for a job or a specific career.

In addition to books, educators can continue to learn and grow in that role through reading a wide variety of journals and/or staying connected with listservs, blogs, websites, or social networking pages that specifically address education issues. **Table 3-1** presents a list of such resources that is by no means an all-encompassing list, but it does point out the variety of resources available to us as educators to learn more about our "craft."

Certainly, another way to continue to develop one's mastery as a teacher is to seek out a mentor or seek help from and dialogue with colleagues who have expertise in education. Think about contacting one of the Fellows in the Academy of Nursing Education, or one of the individuals who participated in the NLN/Johnson & Johnson (J&J) Leadership in Nursing Education Mentor/Protégé Program, or someone who has been inducted into the American Academy of Nursing because of her or his sustained and significant contributions to nursing education. You might also consider contacting an author whose ideas truly "resonate" with your own passions about a mentor relationship or collaboration. Finally, you might consider applying to participate in the NLN/J&J Mentor/Protégé program or the NLN Simulation Fellows program, or any number of other such initiatives, to receive personalized and individualized guidance on your journey toward excellence in nursing education.

As educators, we must continually pursue excellence as teachers, facilitators of learning, pedagogical scholars, educational leaders, and citizens of the academy. This lifelong journey will take us to new

Table 3-1

Selected Education-Focused Journals/Newspapers	
Academic Leader	*International Journal of Nursing*
Action Learning: Research and Practice	*Journal of Curriculum Studies*
American Educational Research Journal	*Journal of Further and Higher Education*
Biomedical Education	*Journal of Multicultural Education*
British Educational Research Journal	*Journal of Nursing Education*
Change (publication of the Carnegie Foundation for the Advancement of Teaching)	*National Forum of Applied Educational Research Journal*
Chronicle of Higher Education	*Nurse Educator*
Community College Journal of Research and Practice	*Nursing Education Perspectives* (National League for Nursing journal)
Comparative and International Education	*Phi Delta Kappan* (journal of Phi Delta Kappa)
Education Policy	*Studies in Higher Education*
Education Media, Technology and Science	*Teacher Education*
Education Scholarship (online)	*Teachers & Teaching*
Educational Action Research	*Teaching in Higher Education*
Educational Researcher	*The Internet and Higher Education*

places, and we will continue to be energized and grow. After all, we are adult learners ourselves!

Summary Thoughts

In this chapter, we have explored various theories of learning and examined how an understanding of the concept of "learning style" can enhance our effectiveness as teachers. We have followed the evolution of the educator role from that of a "sage on the stage" who provides a great deal of information, focuses on the content more so than on the student, and assumes that if something was taught, it also was learned to that of a "guide on the side." The guide challenges students to think deeply, engenders in them a spirit of inquiry, helps them understand who they are as human beings and evolving nurses, and allows them to have more control over the educational experience.

We hope you have been challenged to "do philosophy" and reflect deeply on the insights such self-exploration leads to. Knowing who we are as human beings and what we value will strengthen our ability to guide students on their journey to reach personal and professional goals. It serves to ensure that we do not attempt to "create students in our own image."

Finally, this discussion has outlined the complexity of the educator role and the multiple competencies associated with that role. It is hoped that you have been stimulated to outline a plan for the ongoing development of the knowledge and skills you need as an educator, as well as to consider a scholarly path you might pursue that will enable you to contribute to the evolving science of nursing education.

The nurse educator role and the teaching experience in nursing are both challenging and incredibly rewarding. Do not hesitate to allow your passion for teaching to be evident to students, and do not hesitate to continually question how we can improve the nursing education experience for students and faculty.

Summary Points

1. Such "good citizenship" requires that educators be effective teachers and advisors.

2. Educators also are expected to design, implement and evaluate the curricula in their discipline, taking into account the institution's mission, goals, and degree requirements.

3. Faculty members are responsible for developing, implementing, evaluating, and revising (as needed) policies and procedures related to a number of areas, such as student admission, progression, and graduation; peer review; and tenure and promotion.

4. Educators, however, are something else. They are the individuals whose professional responsibility and major contribution to society relate to enhancing the total development of learners—their minds, their values, their skills—and to advancing knowledge and understanding in their field.

5. Faculty members are challenged to provide learners with problems that challenge them to construct new ideas or concepts—based on what they know and what they seek to find out—that allow them to manage those problems.

6. Learning styles can be thought of as unique ways in which individuals perceive, interact with, process and respond to information and learning situations.

7. In essence, educators need to strive to create learner-centered systems that focus on inquiry, attend to the total development of the learner, actively involve learners, call upon many senses, and challenge learners to think about their thinking.

8. The role of the educator is to facilitate learning, encourage collaboration, help students learn how to learn, empower learners, challenge students to take responsibility for their own learning, and encourage and support a spirit of inquiry.

Tips for Nurse Educators to Use

1. Use a variety of teaching strategies in order to "connect" with the diversity of students and the array of learning styles and intelligences they present.

2. Question the assumptions you make about students and teachers that influence what you do as a teacher.

3. Read extensively about teaching/learning and incorporate new ideas into what you do as a teacher.

4. Ensure that your teaching practices are based on evidence, rather than solely on tradition and past practice.

5. Use a variety of evaluation methods that attend to affective-domain learning, as well as the cognitive and psychomotor domains.

6. Reflect carefully and often on what you do as a teacher and how it can be improved to best serve students. In other words, engage in the scholarship of teaching (Boyer, 1990).

7. Seek out colleagues or mentors with whom you can engage in serious dialogue about teaching, learning, curriculum development, implementing the educator role, and issues in higher education.

8. Allow your passion for teaching to shine for students and faculty colleagues.

References

Atherton, J. S. (2009). *Learning and teaching; Piaget's developmental theory.* Retrieved December 8, 2010, from www.learningandteaching.info/learning/piaget.htm

Bandura, A. (1977). *Social learning theory.* Englewood Cliffs, NJ: Prentice Hall.

Boyer, E.L. (1990). *Scholarship reconsidered: Priorities of the professoriate.* Princeton, NJ: The Carnegie Foundation for the Advancement of Teaching.

Chickering, A. W., & Gamson, Z. F. (1987). Seven principles for good practice in undergraduate education. *The Wingspread Journal, 9*(2), 1−5. Retrieved December 8, 2010, from http://learningcommons.evergreen.edu/pdf/fall1987.pdf

Dewey, J. (1916). *Democracy and education: An introduction to the philosophy of education.* New York: The Free Press.

Gagne, R. M. (1965). *The conditions of learning.* New York, NY: Holt, Reinhart & Winston.

Gardner, H. (1999). *Intelligence reframed: Multiple intelligences for the 21st century.* New York, NY: Basic Books.

Greene, M. (1973). *Teacher as stranger: Educational philosophy in the modern age.* Belmont, CA: Wadsworth.

Gregorc, A. F. (1984). *Gregorc Style Delineator: Development, technical, and administration manual.* Columbia, CT: Gregorc Associates.

Halstead, J. A. (2007). *Nurse educator competencies: Creating an evidence-based practice for nurse educators.* New York, NY: National League for Nursing.

Jensen, E. P. (2008). *Brain-based learning: The new paradigm of teaching* (2nd ed.). Thousand Oaks, CA: Sage Publications.

Knowles, M. S. (1978). *The adult learner: A neglected species* (2nd ed.). Houston: Gulf.

Kolb, D. A. (1984). *Experiential learning: Experience as the source of learning and development.* London: Prentice Hall.

National League for Nursing. (2005). *Core competencies of nurse educators.* New York, NY: Author. Retrieved December 8, 2010, from http://www.nln.org/profdev/pdf/corecompetencies.pdf

Palmer, P. (2007, 10th anniversary edition). *The courage to teach: Exploring the inner landscape of a teacher's life.* San Francisco, CA: Jossey-Bass.

Perry, W. (1970). *Forms of intellectual and ethical development in the college years: A scheme.* New York, NY: Holt, Reinhart & Winston.

Rogers, C. R. (1969). *Freedom to learn.* Columbus, OH: Charles E. Merrill.

Skinner, B. F. (1974). *About behaviorism.* New York, NY: Vintage Books.

Web Links

www.iep.utm.edu: Internet Encyclopedia of Philosophers (search for "educational philosophers").

www.agelesslearner.com/intros/adultlearning.html: How Adults Learn.

www.honolulu.hawaii.edu/intranet/committees/FacDevCom/guidebk/teachtip/adults-2.htm: Principles of Adult Learning.

www.learningandteaching.info/learning/piaget.htm: Piaget's key ideas.

www.carnegiefoundation.org/publications/sub.asp?key=452&subkey=612&printable=true: Shulman, L. S. (2002). Making differences: A table of learning. *Change*, 34(6), 36−44.

www.carnegiefoundation.org/perspectives/index.asp: *Carnegie Perspectives*, an electronic newsletter that offers different ways to think about teaching and learning.

www.carnegiefoundation.org/perspectives/index.asp?key=92: *Carnegie Conversations*, a forum to engage publicly with the authors and readers of *Carnegie Perspectives*.

www.magnapubs.com/newsletters/edutechreport.html: *The Edutech Report*, which provides accurate, practical advice to implement campus technology initiatives.

www.magnapubs.com/newsletters/enewsletters.html: *Faculty Focus*, a free electronic newsletter for those involved with teaching in higher education.

www.informaworld.com: informaWorld is a service that allows you to subscribe to various journals or register to receive email alerts of the tables of contents for specific journals you select, many of which focus on education.

www.merlot.org/merlot/index.htm: MERLOT is a leading-edge, user-centered, searchable collection of peer-reviewed and peer-selected online learning materials for use in higher education, as well as a set of faculty development support services designed to build and sustain online academic communities where faculty, staff, and students from around the world can share their learning materials and pedagogy.

www.masterteacher.com/publication/detail.cfm?Publication_item_number=15: *The Professor in the Classroom* offers a complete program of inservice programs for college faculty members that gives them the strategies and techniques to become master teachers.

www.magnapubs.com/newsletters/teachingprofessor.html: *The Teaching Professor* offers useful information and inspiration to help faculty members in all disciplines teach more effectively. Each issue features summaries and commentary on the latest pedagogical research as well as first-person articles about implementing various teaching strategies.

Multiple Choice Questions

1. Which of the following learning activities would most likely appeal to a student whose strength is Gardner's visual/spatial intelligence?

   A. Study groups, discussion boards, and group projects
   B. Independent work and self-paced activities
   C. Drawing, working with colors and pictures, and puzzles
   D. Reading, writing, and debating

Rationale:

Visual/spatial intelligence refers to an individual's strength in using visual materials to learn (e.g., maps, charts, pictures).

2. Which of the following principles related to learning styles is a correct statement?

   A. Learning styles cannot be determined through any form of measurement.
   B. We teach how we learn.
   C. Knowing one's own learning style interferes with effective learning.
   D. Teachers should use strategies that best match the learning style that is preferred by most students in the class.

Rationale:

Learning styles can be measured, and knowing one's own learning style helps learners use their strengths to enhance learning. Teachers should use a variety of strategies in order to meet the needs of all learners and to ensure that the strategies used are not overly influenced by our own preferences, because we do tend to teach how we learn.

3. Which of the following set of characteristics best describes left-brain thinking?

   A. Sequential, rule-bound, logical
   B. Analytic, tacit, linear
   C. Nonverbal, integrative, emotional
   D. Artistic, parts more important than the whole, synthesis

Rationale:

Characteristics such as artistic, emotional, tacit, and synthesis are characteristics of right-brain thinking.

4. The concrete random learner described by Gregorc prefers a trial-and-error approach, with breakthroughs through intuitive insights. Which of the following learning activities would be least likely to be preferred by this kind of learner?

   A. Independent study
   B. Computer games and simulations
   C. Model development
   D. Lecture

Rationale:

The concrete random learner likes a stimulus-rich environment and thrives on competition. A lecture would not engage this learner to the extent the other activities would.

5. Which of the following is the most significant "driving force" when deciding what learning activities to design to facilitate student learning?
    A. Students' learning styles
    B. Teacher's learning style
    C. Learning objectives
    D. Experience with using a particular activity

Rationale:

The goals or objectives of a learning experience are the most important factors that guide the development or selection of teaching strategies. Many other factors (such as those noted in the options above) can and should be taken into consideration, but the goals of learning must take priority.

6. Which of the following statements is most closely aligned with the perspectives on teaching and learning expressed by John Dewey?
    A. Learners are motivated by intrinsic goals and the opportunity to learn through discovery.
    B. Learners are motivated by rewards, reinforcement, and punishment.
    C. Advancement in one's cognitive development occurs through being challenged with thinking that is one stage higher than one's current position.
    D. Individuals learn through observing others and what they do.

Rationale:

Rewards and punishment reflect Skinner's perspectives, one-plus stage challenging reflects Perry's model, and social learning is congruent with Bandura's theory. Dewey's perspective promotes intrinsic goal motivation and discovery.

7. Currently, the term *pedagogy* is most closely aligned with which of the following statements?
    A. Teaching should be learner-directed and focus on "the tasks of life."
    B. Learners are passive and subject matter is central.
    C. Teaching is both an art and a science.
    D. Teachers should encourage cooperation among students.

Rationale:

Pedagogy no longer refers to the teaching of children, but to the art and science of teaching.

8. Which of the following *Principles of Good Practice in Undergraduate Education* (Chickering & Gamson, 1987) is identified as the most important factor in engaging students with the material to be studied and facilitate their learning?

    A. Give prompt feedback.
    B. Communicate high expectations.
    C. Encourage cooperation among students.
    D. Encourage student–faculty contact.

    Rationale:

    Though the first three responses are among the *Principles*, the authors note that research indicates that student–faculty contact is the most significant factor in engaging students.

9. When an educator "does philosophy" (Greene, 1973), he or she takes the risk of doing which of the following?

    A. Receiving less-than-positive feedback from peers.
    B. Discovering that what we say we value as teachers is not always congruent with what we do in that role.
    C. Failing when a new teaching approach is used.
    D. Preparing students who are unable to pass the licensing examination.

    Rationale:

    "Doing philosophy" is an introspective process that leads us to think carefully about who we are, what "drives" us, and whether our actions/behaviors match our words or expressed values.

10. Which of the following is *not* a nurse educator competency articulated by the National League for Nursing (2005)?

    A. Function as a change agent and leader.
    B. Maintain certification in a clinical specialization.
    C. Engage in scholarship.
    D. Use assessment and evaluation strategies.

    Rationale:

    The NLN's list of nurse educator competencies notes that the individual pursues continuous quality improvement in the nurse educator role, which may include maintaining some level of expertise and/or certification in a clinical specialty area, but the NLN does not specify that such certification is essential for all nurse educators.

Discussion Questions

1. Who is the "adult learner"? How do approaches to teaching need to be modified when dealing with an adult learner population?

Considerations:

Adult learners are self-directed, goal oriented, problem oriented, and want learning to be relevant. Learning experiences designed by the teacher should encourage students to draw on their past experiences to solve new problems, and the problems presented should be "real-life" challenges so they have relevance.

2. Which theories of learning are most congruent with your own philosophy of education? Which are most incongruent? Which of those theories do you think have (or would have) the greatest influence on you as a teacher?

Considerations:

Highlight major themes of various learning theories. Thoughtfully reflect on their meaning and which are most closely aligned with your own philosophy. Discuss how a learning theory influences the role of the learner, the role of the teacher, the teaching strategies used, learner/ teacher relationships, the nature of the learning environment, and the evaluation methods used.

3. Given that a teacher may know individual students' learning styles, is it possible to accommodate those individual preferences when that teacher is involved with many students during the course of a semester or program? If so, how can you avoid teacher "burnout"? If not, what's all the "fuss" about learning styles, and why bother to find out what they are?

Considerations:

Summarize the major learning styles. Discuss identification of learning styles through self-assessment, completion of tools/instruments, or dialogue and reflection with others (e.g., the teacher). Discuss the usefulness of knowing one's style to "play to one's strengths." Consider the need to match teaching strategies and learning experiences with learning goals, more so than with learning styles.

4. Some assert that nursing faculty want students to be humanistic with patients, yet they themselves are behavioristic with students. What do the two perspectives mean in the context of education, and why might this phenomenon occur in nursing?

Considerations:

Reflect on the meaning of humanism and behaviorism in the context of education. Develop insights regarding the realities of nursing education (e.g., licensure examination, accreditation standards, etc.).

5. Choose *one* of the following quotes and reflect on its meaning. For the T. S. Eliot quote, think about how it relates to "doing educational philosophy." For the Tosteson quote, think about what it means to how you implement your role as an educator.

> **T. S. Eliot:** *We shall not cease from exploration. And the end of all our exploring will be to arrive where we started and know the place for the first time.*

> **Tosteson:** *We must acknowledge again that the most important, indeed, the only thing we have to offer our students is ourselves. Everything else they can read in a book or discover independently, usually with a better understanding than our efforts can convey.*

Considerations:

Consider how "doing philosophy" challenges us to reflect on who we are, what we believe, and what our actions truly convey about how we perceive others. As a result of such introspection, we come to know ourselves, look at others, and perceive situations in new ways. Consider how reflecting on "what we have to offer students" challenges educators to think about the significance of their role and how everything they say and do (or fail to say or fail to do) sends a message to students, thereby influencing them. The educator role is, indeed, a potentially most powerful one.

Teaching Scenario

Judy Mack is a new faculty member who has been assigned to teach a lower-division (i.e., freshman or sophomore year) course on health assessment at a nearby baccalaureate nursing program. She must teach the theory/lab course within the framework of the approved course objectives, but otherwise she has the freedom to develop the course in any way she sees fit. Judy is excited about the possibilities this course presents and wants to implement all of what she learned in graduate school about teaching and learning.

The sophomore students who will be enrolling in the course have completed a one-credit "Introduction to Nursing as Profession" course as freshmen as well as foundational courses in the biological and social sciences. Judy realizes that each of the 30 students in her class has developed her or his own approach to learning, and she is hopeful that she can satisfy everyone's needs, including her own.

■ How can Judy identify each student's learning style without using large amounts of class time?

■ What learning styles should Judy expect to find among this student group that ranges in age from 19 to 52 and includes males and females, several students whose basic education was completed outside the United States, and students who have transferred to this school from another nursing program?

Judy decides to structure the course as follows: lecture on one aspect of assessment on Monday, demonstrate it in lab on Wednesday, remind students of the hours the lab will be open for them to practice the assessment, and test them on that aspect of assessment the following Wednesday in lab. She is careful to correlate the class session with the "Anatomy and Physiology" content the students are learning simultaneously and is patient in answering individual students' questions about how this assessment knowledge will help their nursing practice.

■ What learning principles has Judy applied appropriately?

■ What learning principles has Judy violated?

■ How could Judy better structure this course to fulfill more principles of learning and meet a wider array of learning styles/preferences?

Judy has now been asked to teach a similar course for RNs through the school's continuing education department.

■ What modifications should Judy make in the course, given this particular learner population?

■ What principles of adult learning are evidenced by these modifications?

Bibliography

Amerson, R. (2006). Energizing the nursing lecture: Application of the theory of multiple intelligence learning. *Nursing Education Perspectives, 27*(4), 194–203.

Ard, N. (2009). Essentials of learning. In C. M. Shultz (Ed.), *Building a science of nursing education: Foundations for evidence-based teaching/learning* (pp. 25–131). New York, NY: National League for Nursing.

Ashley, J. A., & LaBelle, B. M. (1976). Education for freeing minds. In J. A. Williamson (Ed.), *Current perspectives in nursing education—The changing scene* (Vol. I, pp. 50–65). St. Louis: Mosby.

Carter, S. L. (1978). The nurse educator: Humanist or behaviorist? *Nursing Outlook, 26*(9), 554–557.

Coffield, F., Moseley, D., Hall, E., & Ecclestone, K. (2004). Learning styles and pedagogy in post-16 learning: A systematic and critical review. Retrieved December 8, 2010, from http://www.pedagogy.ir/index.php?option=com_content&view=article&id=140:learning-styles-and-pedagogy-in-post-16-learning-a-systematic-and-critical-review&catid=47:constructivism&Itemid=71

Eliot, T. S. Retrieved on November 13, 2010 from http://www.brainyquote.com/quotes/quotes/t/tseliot109032.html

Glenn, D. (2009, December 16). Matching teaching style to learning style may not help students. *Chronicle of Higher Education.*

Greer, A.G., Pokorny, M., Clay, M.C., Brown, S., & Steele, L. L. (2010). Learner-centered characteristics of nurse educators. *International Journal of Nursing Education Scholarship, 7*(1), Article 6.

Hartley, M. P. (2010). Experiential learning using Kolb's cycle of learning [Syllabus Selection]. *Journal of Nursing Education, 49*(2), 120.

Honigsfeld, A., & Dunn, R. (2006, Winter). Learning-style characteristics of adult learners. *The Delta Kappa Gamma Bulletin, 14–17*, 31.

Jewell, M. L. (1994). Partnership in learning: Education as liberation. *Nursing & Health Care, 15*(7), 360–364.

Kohlberg, L., & Mayer, R. (1972). Development as the aim of education. *Harvard Educational Review, 42*(4), 449–496.

Kostovich, C., Poradzisz, M., Wood, K., & O'Brien, K. L. (2007). Learning style preference and student aptitude for concept maps. *Journal of Nursing Education, 46*(5), 225–231.

McDaniels, O. B. (1983). Existentialism and pragmatism: The effect of philosophy on methodology of teaching. *Journal of Nursing Education, 22*(2), 62–66.

Philosophy of teaching statements: Examples and tips on how to write a teaching philosophy statement. (2009). *Faculty Focus,* Special Report, May 2009. Madison, WI: Magna Publications.

Robinson, F. P. (2009). Servant teaching: The power and promise for nursing education. *International Journal of Nursing Education Scholarship, 6*(1), Article 5.

Smoyak, S. A. (1978). Teaching as coaching. *Nursing Education, 26*(6), 361–363.

Tabak, N., Adi, L., & Eherenfeld, M. (2003). A philosophy underlying excellence in teaching. *Nursing Philosophy, 4*, 249–254.

Thompson, C., & Crutchlow, E. (1993). Learning style research: A critical review of the literature and implications for nursing education. *Journal of Professional Nursing, 9*(1), 34–40.

Tosteson, D. C. (1979). Learning in medicine. *New England Journal of Medicine, 301* (13), 690–694.

Other Resource

Tomorrow's Professor is an electronic resource that is available at no cost. Every few days, you will receive an email that gives a summary of a book, article, presentation, or other resource related to education, teaching and learning, faculty roles, and so forth. You can subscribe to the Tomorrow's-Professor Mailing List by sending the message [subscribe tomorrows-professor] to: Majordomo@lists. stanford.edu.

Chapter 4

Ethics in Teaching

Sharon Cannon and Carol Boswell

Chapter Objectives

At the conclusion of this chapter, the learner will be able to:

1. Discuss policies impacted by legislative and regulatory agencies.
2. Distinguish the differences in HIPAA and FERPA in relation to ethics in nursing education.
3. Discuss ethics.
4. Discuss ethical issues in teaching in higher education.

Key Terms

- ➤ Care ethics
- ➤ Commission on Collegiate Nursing Education
- ➤ Deontology
- ➤ Ethics
- ➤ FERPA
- ➤ HIPAA
- ➤ Joint Commission

- ➤ Legislative policy
- ➤ National League for Nursing Accrediting Commission
- ➤ Regulatory policy
- ➤ Rights ethical theory
- ➤ Utilitarianism
- ➤ Virtue ethical theory

Introduction

Nurses and nurse educators are challenged daily by legal and ethical considerations in their practice. Nurse educators are in a unique position of having to balance legal/ethical issues from two perspectives, as a nurse and as a nurse educator. The two are intertwined and yet, at times, are separate. There are legal/ethical issues unique, yet similar, to each, such as laws that govern the release of student's grades to parents and the restriction of patient information to families. The only similarity in this example is release of information, but the actual laws and ethics for each are different in the enactment, audience, and setting. The nurse at the bedside does not need to know the information disclosure law for students, but the nurse educator must be cognizant of both.

To fully understand the relationship of ethics to legal aspects of nursing and nursing education, a definition of each is in order. Sumner (2011) indicated that the term **ethics** comes from the Greek word *ethos* and reflects societal standards. The term *legal* pertains to laws which are established by society. Keep in mind that though primitive societies such as remote tribes in South America can differ greatly from a population such as in the United States, each has norms for standards of behavior. Violations in either society bring repercussions for unacceptable behaviors. Aiken (2004) states that "ethics are declarations of what is right or wrong and what ought to be" (p. 100). Regardless of societal sophistication, there are governing bodies and guidelines relating to acceptable behavior. In nursing and nursing education, legal and ethical standards guide nursing practice and education.

Legislative and Regulatory Policy

Many nurses, regardless of their practice setting, equate legislation with politics, and thus ignore the huge impact that legislation has upon their practice. Sad to say, but the fact that few nurses are informed voters (if they vote at all) is common knowledge. Boswell, Cannon, and Miller (2005) suggested political involvement is a responsibility, not a privilege. Laws (**legislative policy**) and regulations (**regulatory policy**) are embedded in nursing practice and nursing education. Laws come from city, county, state, and national policy. Rules and regulations follow the same path by establishing guidelines based upon laws. Both have governing bodies to carry out the required standard. In addition, professions such as medicine, nursing, pharmacy, and so forth have codes of ethics and governing bodies to regulate the profession. For example, many national nursing organizations have a code of ethics that involves doing no harm to patients under nursing care. State Boards of Nursing, whose sole purpose is to protect patients, are present to regulate nursing practice and nursing education. To further comprehend legislative/regulatory policies and their interactions in nursing education, an examination of two legislative acts is necessary.

HIPAA and FERPA

The Health Insurance Portability and Accountability Act (**HIPAA**) was enacted in 1996 to protect health information through a "privacy rule" to establish standards about the use and disclosure of health information (Department of Health and Human Services, n.d.). The final form of the Privacy Rule was published in 2002. HIPAA determines:

1. who is covered,
2. what information is protected,
3. principles for use and disclosure,
4. permitted use and disclosure,
5. authorized uses and disclosure,
6. limiting uses and disclosures to the minimum necessary,
7. notice and other individual rights,
8. administrative requirements,
9. organizational options,
10. personal representative and minors,
11. state laws,
12. enforcement and penalties for noncompliance, and
13. compliance dates.

Obviously, HIPAA has huge implications for nurses and has become more complex with the advent of new methods of communication, especially computer technology such as emails, iPods, texting, and blogs. Communication is no longer limited to what is faxed or talked about in the hallways and elevators, but has expanded through technology to include multiple new modalities. This affects the nurse educator in the areas of developing case studies, conducting pre- and post clinical conferences, creating care plans, reviewing student logs/journals and student papers, conducting simulation lab scenarios, and giving lectures, to name just a few. Care must be taken that patient identification is not apparent regardless of the instructional methodology employed in the classroom, clinical setting, or online courses.

The Family Educational Rights and Privacy Act (**FERPA**) was enacted in 1974 and is commonly known as the Buckley Amendment. This law protects the privacy of student education records, and applies to all schools receiving federal funds. Prior to the age of 18, a student's parents have the right to their child's education records. After the age of 18, the rights transfer to the student (Department of Education, n.d.). FERPA spells out:

1. who is eligible to receive information,
2. how to correct inaccurate or misleading information,
3. how student information can be released,
4. the type of information that may be disclosed without consent,
5. notification about directory information with allowances for a nondisclosure
6. request, and annual notification of rights under FERPA.

FERPA appears simple but is extremely complex and far reaching. The use of the Internet, external regulations, and accrediting bodies all play a major role in how FERPA affects students. Guidelines state where and how grades can be posted. For instance, posting grades on a bulletin board outside a faculty member's office isn't allowed. In addition, use of a student's identification number or social security number is a violation.

Faculty actions must be based on legally sanctioned facts. Faculty are being compared to national standards rather than the prior "locality rules" (Gumby, 2008). In other words, faculty members cannot act on whether or not they like a student, or claim that the local norm allows faculty members to act in contradiction to standards set by national organizations/agencies.

Faculty, as well as students, can be held accountable for clinical negligence. "Do no harm" to patients can also be extended to faculty to protect students from harm related to exposure to violence and needle sticks. Another consideration that has changed over the years is that students do not practice under their faculty's nursing licensure, and faculty may need to intervene to protect the patients.

In addition, FERPA has implications for students with disabilities. In this instance, the student must provide evidence and documentation of the disability with proposed accommodations. Caution is advised here depending on the disability and requirements necessary to complete assignments in the clinical setting. Faculty and school administrators must work to effectively manage those disabilities which are documented. Some examples of the different means which have been used are: (1) longer time periods to complete examinations, (2) readers for those individuals who are hearing impaired, and (3) computers provided for those with physical disabilities.

As in all education systems, policies and procedures must exist to allow students due process for academic dishonesty, failing grades, and being unsafe in clinical settings. HIPAA and FERPA apply to both students and patients. A school's policies and procedures must incorporate all rights for both students and their patients.

Regulatory Agencies

Accreditation will be addressed in Chapter 9, but its influence on the education of nurses and the faculty role must be mentioned at this point. The **Joint Commission** accredits healthcare organizations and sets standards required for consumers of health care, especially hospitals and clinics where nurses are employed. Thus, faculty members are required to maintain competence in nursing practice to be able to teach students in these settings. Without accreditation, hospitals are ineligible for federal funds and are often not financially viable, thus lacking high standards of care. There are several educational organizations that set standards for higher education institutions. They are organized by region and are designated as a commission, such as the Commission on Colleges of the Southern Association of Colleges and Schools or the Northwest Commission on Colleges and Universities. These commissions accredit colleges and universities that have schools of nursing. Colleges and universities without accreditation are also ineligible for federal funds, especially for Pell Grants, traineeships, and so forth, which can result in students being unable to afford an education in nursing.

Schools of Nursing are also accredited by two national nursing organizations. The National League for Nursing (NLN) accredits all nursing programs through the **National League for Nursing Accrediting Commission** (NLNAC). The American Association of Colleges of Nursing (AACN) provides accreditation for baccalaureate and graduate nursing programs through the **Commission on Collegiate Nursing Education** (CCNE)

The two most important regulatory agencies for nursing are the National Council of State Boards of Nursing (NCSBN) and each state, commonwealth, and/or territorial's board of nursing. The NCSBN's purpose is "to ensure public protection, each jurisdiction requires candidates for licensure to pass an examination that measures the competencies needed to perform safely and effectively as a newly licensed entry-level registered nurse" (NCSBN, n.d., p. 3 of 10).

The second regulatory agency is each state's Board of Nursing (BON). State BONs are to protect and promote the welfare of its citizens. Unfortunately, many nurses think that their BON is for nurses, but it is not; BONs regulate the practice of nursing and the approval of nursing education programs. Each state has laws with rules and regulations for the practice of nursing, and is often derived from the

Nursing Practice Act of the state. The services of BONs range from licensing school approval to enforcement of laws to provision of information. Faculty members must have a current, valid license to practice nursing and the appropriate education credentials to teach nursing.

As can be seen, legislative/regulatory agencies, HIPAA, and FERPA, along with accrediting bodies, are integral to the role of faculty. Each of these affects ethical issues in higher education regarding the practice of nursing and the teaching of nursing.

Ethics

According to Rainbow (2002), "ethical theories and principles are the foundation of ethical analysis because they are the viewpoints from which guidance can be obtained along the pathway to a decision" (para. 1). When ethics is used effectively, decisions are based upon specific guidelines and information. The different ethical theories and principles provide the societal standards on which decisions can be made. O'Connor (2010) states that "learning to acknowledge personal moral views, to analyze and evaluate moral opinions, to reflect on moral situations, to defend moral choices, and to work with other healthcare team members on resolutions of ethical/moral situations and dilemmas is critical to the development of the ethical nurse" (p. 621). Nurses and nurse educators must accept the responsibility for incorporating personal moral views, opinions, situations, and choices into the day-to-day experiences of peers and students. All aspects within the delivery of health care are transformed by an understanding and acknowledgement of the moral/ethical obligations which the nursing profession embraces.

Nelson (2003) further supports these ideas because the ethical principles which provide the foundation for ethical decision making are founded upon moral values. These subtle moral ideals are not enforceable by any laws. The principles subsumed within ethical decisions are not laws in and of themselves, but are the foundational components which guide the behaviors used when confronted by situations outside the control of laws. The six major ethical principles are: autonomy, veracity, nonmalfeasance, confidentiality, beneficence, and justice. Each of these tenets is used to maneuver toward an outcome when a situation is not covered by legal precedents.

As one begins to investigate the different principles foundational for ethical decisions, the first one to be considered is autonomy. According to Nelson (2003), autonomy is related to the idea that each of us has the right to self-determine the aspects within our lives. Laws have been established to protect the ability for individuals to choose independently concerning situations encountered. Each person is understood to have the right and responsibly to make free choices about the decisions that are key to their private lives. The independent control over individual existence is held as a critical principle for the uniqueness of each person. Rainbow (2002) states that "each man deserves respect, because only he has had those exact life experiences and understands his emotions, motivations, and body in such an intimate manner" (para. 5). These emotions, motivations, and life experiences shape how an individual comes to the unique decisions encountered in the ethical dimension. Within the principles of autonomy, each individual is allowed to pull from his or her culture and environment when making those decisions not addressed by legal rules.

A second principle of ethical decision making is the concept of veracity. Veracity is understood to represent truth telling. The confines of ethical decisions are closely linked with informed decision making and informed consent (Nelson, 2003). For each decision with which a person is confronted, the expectation is that truthful information will be provided by all involved parties, so the affected individual can use the entirety of the information to make the appropriate decision. All decisions rest upon the idea that the individuals involved in the determination have all of the necessary information to make a full and complete decision about the situation encountered. Without factual and complete information, the effectiveness of the decision-making process is compromised.

Another tenet in ethical decision making is the concept of non-malfeasance. This is a busy term that basically means "do no harm." Within health care particularly, the idea of doing no harm to individuals is paramount. This principle of not harming someone is foundational in ethical aspects and is vital to the fabric of legal determination. Nonmalfeasance is one of the key aspects when negligence and/or malpractice issues are raised. According to Rainbow (2002), individuals could "reasonably argue that people have a greater responsibility to 'do no harm' than to take steps to benefit others" (para. 4). Someone who chooses to harm a person tends to be directly in opposition to the fabric of societal standards. In all situations, the expectations is that individuals will endeavor to not harm others. Though this aspect is not always possible, the thought is that in all situations the push is to not do any harm, or at least as little harm as possible.

A fourth principle used for ethical decision making is the idea of confidentiality. Confidentiality is viewed as the securing of all privileged information which is obtained as a result of professional capacity with a patient or client. In each and every situation, the maintaining of private information in a secure and protected manner is viewed as the standard. Materials and/or information gained as a consequence of providing care to an individual is considered to be privileged communication. For all information controlled due to the manner or setting in which it was collected, the protection and privacy of the information must be closely guarded. Within the arena of ethical decision making, the materials gained from this type of discussion remain the sole property of the patient and/or client.

Another aspect of ethical decision making is the concept of beneficence. Frequently, this component is viewed as "doing good." Rainbow (2002) states that "this principle stipulates that ethical theories should strive to achieve the greatest amount of good because people benefit from the most good" (para. 2). For each and every situation, the focus is expected to be on the actions that will bring about the greatest good or most beneficial outcome for those involved.

The final principle subsumed under ethical decision making is the idea of justice. Justice is viewed as the fairness of the situation. This concept entails striving to ensure equality for all individuals in regard to goods, services, and protection. Consistency within the determination of decisions for each and every individual is the mindset when considering a decision to be founded on justice. The formation of decisions based upon a consistent logical foundation on which to resolve the ethical situation under consideration is imperative and essential.

After carefully considering the foundational principles utilized within ethical theories, a discussion of the different ethical theories can be undertaken. Books have been written on the different ethical theories; thus, an in-depth dialogue concerning these theories is outside the scope of this chapter. An overview of the different theories will be provided: deontology, utilitarianism, virtue ethics, care ethics, and rights ethics. Each of these theories considers the ethical situation from a different approach, resulting in discrete management of the state of affairs.

Deontology for ethical considerations is founded on rules. Deontological theory obliges the addressing of any ethical situation based on the idea that correctness originates from rules and duty (O'Connor, 2010; Rainbow, 2002). The upholding of a person's obligation is the foundation on which this theory is based. The rules, regulations, standards, and/or policies are the underpinning for all decisions related to ethical situations. Rainbow (2002) states that a person utilizing this theory "will produce very consistent decisions since they will be based on the individual's set duties" (para. 10). Though the strength of this theory is the steadiness and reliability of the resulting management of ethical situations, the challenge relates to the requirement of implementing the rules without a consideration for the welfare of those involved. The entire focus for this theory is the use of those selected rules in a consistent manner. Within the use of this theory, the rules, regulations, standards, and/or policies are expected to be established on what is best for the individuals involved. Thus when the foundation of rules is based upon this concept, the application of the rules should benefit those involved.

The second theory used within ethical decision making is **utilitarianism**. It is also called the consequentialist, teleology, or situation theory (Aiken, 2004). This theory is based upon outcomes. The decisions made using this theory would endeavor to envision the consequences of each action possible. As a result of considering all of the possible outcomes, the best decision for the most individuals can be selected. This theory works to provide the solution which prompts the maximum advantage for the majority of the people involved in the situation. Within this theory, the focus can be directed in two different directions. One is the act of utilitarianism which omits personal feelings or societal constraints when making the decision. This type of outcome is based on the benefit to the most individual without considering any other aspect. The other focus is called rule utilitarianism. For this focus, laws and fairness are utilized when the decision is being made. Fairness and justice are viewed as foundational in this focus, and these concepts are used to help determine the solution that will benefit the majority of the individuals involved. The primary concern when using utilitarianism as a method for decision making is the aspect of effectively predicting outcomes. This predicting of outcomes requires that the decisions be made based on knowledge of the future. The need to foresee into the future is a flaw of this theory.

The **virtue ethical theory** has grown in support and functionality over the last few years. According to O'Connor (2010), "virtue ethics focuses on the traits of good character that individuals develop over years, influenced by family, faith communities, education, and society" (p. 627). The foundation for this theory is character rather than actions or rules. The character of a person in normal behavior is used as the groundwork for determining the plan for managing an ethical situation. One of the primary concerns ensuing from this theory relates to the changing views of "normal" behavior. As individuals encounter different situations and learning opportunities, their behaviors frequently reflect the evolving knowledge and culture. With every change in behavior, prior ethical decisions are then called into question, as they were based on "normal" behavior at that time. Normal behavior can be significantly modified as societal aspects change. Another concern with the use of this theory is the problem encountered when an individual is labeled by society as not engaging in "normal" accepted behavior. The labeling of individuals becomes the problem, not necessarily the behavior being used within the decision-making process. A person can demonstrate both normal and abnormal behaviors reflective of a specific setting. For this theory, the behavior used at the time of the decision-making process is the criterion for the decision.

A fourth ethical theory which can be used in the decision-making process is the **rights ethical theory**. In this theory, rights as established by society and endorsed by the larger, ruling population are used as the foundation for the decisions made. As long as the rights set forth by this population are ethically correct, the decisions resulting from the decisions will be ethical in nature. The determination of the societal rights becomes a key aspect when utilizing this theory.

The final ethical theory for consideration is **care ethics**. According to O'Connor (2010), this theory centers on the interaction of the specific nurse and the individual patient or family. As an individual uses this process, the participants are expected to contemplate the milieu of the circumstances, preserve the interactions involving the individuals, and ensure that everyone is supported and strengthened. Within the care theory of ethics, the persons involved in the decision are key to the determination of the action plan to be enforced. Only when everyone is in agreement with the direction to be taken is the situation effectively managed. One grave problem with this theory is the realization that getting everyone to agree to a plan of action is sometimes very difficult, if not impossible.

Ethical situations provide everyone with the opportunities to grow and develop. At times, it is difficult and frustrating. Since ethical standards are based upon a moral foundation, the stressors involved frequently become personal in nature. Each participant in the decision-making process comes to the table with different moral backgrounds. Individuals can move on several different paths toward a goal or outcome based upon those principles and theories used within the decision-making process.

Ethics of Teaching in Higher Education

As we move from general consideration of ethical aspects to their application to teaching, several different thoughts and challenges become evident. Nurses at the bedside deal with ethical situations which tend to relate to the physical side of their professional practice. Life, death, quality of life, quantity of life, informed consent, privacy/confidentiality, and other aspects tend to be the focus for ethical situations which tend to impact the physical care of the client. Ethics within the teaching realm moves toward the management of individuals. Usually in the teaching realm, faculty members do not worry about whether their students are going to live or die. It is more about the moral development of the individual instead of the physical management of the individual. Thus, the application moves to the determination and application of the moral behaviors resulting in the clarification of a decision.

Each of the six principles within ethics is critical when considering both the HIPAA and FERPA aspects within the educational process. Since both of these laws tend to deal more with information, the principles of veracity, confidentiality, and justice are highly important within the finalization of a decision. Having acknowledged the importance of these three does not negate the contributions of autonomy, nonmalfeasance, and beneficence. Faculty members and school administrators must constantly remember that each student is unique. Though the rules and regulations can be used to ensure nonmalfeasance and beneficence in the management of the educational environment, each student comes with a unique history which must be carefully considered when addressing the different aspects controlled by HIPAA and FERPA regulations.

According to O'Connor (2010), "teaching ethics is an important area that can be used as an area of content to emphasize the importance of attitude and fair thinking" (p. 620). The teaching and utilization of ethical principles within the classroom/clinical experience serves to serendipitously reinforce the students' capacity to distinguish individual values, to critically cogitate, to act as a team, and to evade any violation of academic integrity, such as plagiarism. Faculty members can provide these opportunities in many ways. Condon (2008) stated that "one's ethics provides the grounds for every action taken or not taken in relation to students and faculty colleagues" (p. 402). Some examples of showcasing ethical behavior are: (1) acting as an ethical role model as decisions are made, (2) using student discussion groups to struggle with ethical dilemmas, (3) facilitating values-clarification activities to allow students to safely investigate their values, and (4) using case studies that incorporate ethical principles in the management of the scenario. Providing safe environments where the students can dissect the ethical situations and arrive at alternative decisions allows the students to test out conduits for use when they are confronted with similar situations in less structured settings. The American Nurses Association (ANA) in 2001 revised and updated the *Code of Ethics for Nurses with Interpretive Statements*. This document provides a universal foundation used by American nurses as they work within an ethical framework. Though we do not at this time have a unique code for nurse educators, the ethical principles maintained within the ANA code provide an underpinning which is acceptable in practice and educational settings. The International Council of Nurses (ICN) also has a Code of Ethics for Nursing (approved 2000). Within this code, the expectations of ethical behavior are presented with an international focus. A code of ethics is a "written list of a profession's values and standards of conduct" (Aiken, 2004, p. 100). Such codes form the pedestal on which a profession practices. The aspects noted within a code of ethics do not provide specific examples but do provide the values and expectations by which the professionals are expected to function.

Tippitt, Ard, Kline, Tilghman, Chamberlain, and Meagher (2009) presented several interesting thoughts related to ethics and academic integrity. Within their article, academic integrity was defined as "a commitment, even in the face of adversity, to five fundamental values: honesty, trust, fairness, respect, and responsibility" (Tippitt et al., 2009, para. 2). Since academic integrity is a key aspect of ethical behavior within higher education, it becomes very important that faculty members provide an effective role modeling of the practices which reflect integrity. Some of the questions suggested by this article to focus a faculty member's thought toward academic integrity are:

1. Does the academic institution itself demonstrate a culture of academic integrity?
2. Are rules/policies created for the sake of having them, or do faculty and administrators explain the rationale for policies to students and faculty?
3. Does the curriculum lend itself to integrity?
4. Are the objectives for assignments clear?
5. Are assignments being given as busywork, or do they facilitate significant learning?
6. Are specific program outcomes in place related to the affective domain, such as honesty, integrity, and values?
7. How do faculty model and mentor students in acquiring and living within these values? (Tippitt et al., 2009, paras. 10–12)

As faculty members strive to apply the ideas of ethical decision making and academic integrity to the educational setting, several strategies can be employed to diminish or avert academic misconduct, such as assigning seats for students, jumbling up the order of the test questions, restricting the things students are allowed to have available during an exam, and having all examinations proctored. Though these strategies are effective in reducing the potential for academic misconduct, they are frequently viewed as negative in nature. These strategies seek to prevent students from engaging in problematic behavior, which implies that faculty members expect students to engage in academic misconduct. Using strategies that showcase the expectation that students should not participate in academic misconduct sets up a positive and supportive environment for learning.

Summary Thoughts

Ethical issues are all around us within the academic arena and the health arena. As faculty members, it becomes vital and essential for each of us to carefully consider the message we are providing in regard to ethics. Each faculty member must develop a firm foundation related to key legislative and regulatory policies such as HIPAA and FERPA. In addition to this underpinning, nursing faculty members must also be very aware of the different codes of ethics of the nursing and education professions. O'Connor (2010) stated that "faculty members must be prepared to facilitate thinking about ethics in their students by acting as ethical persons of integrity both personally and professionally" (p. 621). As faculty members, it is our responsibility to present an effective role model for ethical behavior based upon a firm understanding of legislative and regulatory policies. To demonstrate any less is to provide the example that ethics is not an integral part of effective health and educational practices.

Summary Points

1. The term *ethics* comes from the Greek word *ethos* and reflects societal standards.
2. When using ethics effectively, decisions are based upon specific guidelines and information. The different ethical theories and principles provide the societal standards on which decisions can be made.
3. All aspects within the delivery of health care are transformed by an understanding and acknowledgement of the moral/ethical obligations which the nursing profession embraces.
4. The independent control over individual existence is held as a critical principle for the uniqueness of each person.
5. Deontological theory obliges the addressing of any situation based on the idea that correctness originates from rules and duty.
6. Utilitarianism theory endeavors to envision the consequences of each action possible.
7. The virtue ethical theory focuses on the aspects of good character.
8. Rights ethical theory uses rights established by society and endorsed by the larger, ruling population.
9. Care ethical theory centers on the interaction of the specific nurse and the individual patient or family.

10. Legislative and regulatory policies are embedded in nursing practice.
11. The Health Insurance Portability and Accountability Act (HIPAA) was enacted in 1996 to protect health information.
12. The Family Educational Rights and Privacy Act (FERPA) was enacted in 1974 to protect the privacy of students.
13. Both HIPAA and FERPA have implications for teaching nursing.
14. Educational accrediting commissions and the Joint Commission have standards governing nursing educational programs and the practice of nursing.
15. The National League of Nursing (NLN) and the American Association of Colleges of Nursing (AACN) accredit programs of nursing.
16. The National Council of State Boards of Nursing (NCSBN) and state Boards of Nursing (BONs) have as their mission to protect the welfare of the public.
17. The NCSBN developed a test to measure competence needed to perform safely and effectively as a newly licensed, entry-level registered nurse, regardless of state, commonwealth, or territory of the United States.
18. State BONs regulate the practice of nursing and approval of nursing education programs.
19. Ethics within the teaching realm moves toward the management of individuals.
20. The teaching and utilization of ethical principles within the classroom/clinical experience serves to serendipitously reinforce the students' capacity to distinguish individual values, to critically cogitate, to act as a team, and to evade any violation of academic integrity, such as plagiarism.
21. Using strategies that showcase the expectation that students should not participate in academic misconduct sets up a positive and supportive environment for learning.

Tips for Nurse Educators to Use

1. The nurse educator must be politically active to be an advocate for students, patients, and the nursing profession.
2. Having a solid foundation of HIPAA and FERPA policies enhances the effectiveness of nursing faculty.
3. Legislative/regulatory agencies mandate standards by which nurse educators must abide.
4. The NCSBN and the state BONs are concerned with the competence of entry-level registered nurses and the safety of the public.
5. Accrediting agencies for health care and higher education promote quality outcomes for patients and students.
6. Ethical and moral development involve the determination and application of moral behaviors within the clarification of a decision.

7. Some examples for showcasing ethical behavior are: (1) acting as an ethical role model as decisions are made, (2) using student discussion groups to struggle with ethical dilemmas, (3) facilitating values-clarification activities to allow students to safely investigate their values, and (4) providing case studies that incorporate ethical principles in the management of the scenario.

8. Several strategies can be employed to diminish or avert academic misconduct, such as assigning seats for students, jumbling up the order of the test questions, restricting the things students are allowed to have available during an exam, and having all examinations proctored.

References

Aiken, T. D. (2004). *Legal, ethical, and political issues in nursing* (2nd ed.). Philadelphia, PA: F.A. Davis Company.

Boswell, C., Cannon, S., & Miller, J. (2005). Nurses' political involvement: Responsibility versus privilege. *Journal of Professional Nursing*, 21(1), 5–8.

Condon, E. H. (2008). Ethical issues in teaching nursing. In B. K. Penn (Ed.), *Mastering the teaching role: A guide for nurse educators* (Chapter 30). Philadelphia, PA: F.A. Davis Company.

Department of Education. (n.d.). Family educational rights and privacy act. Retrieved January 4, 2010, from http://www.edu.gov/policy/gen/guide/fpco/ferpa/index.html

Department of Human Health Services. (n.d.). Health Insurance Portability and Accountability Act. Retrieved January 4, 2010, from http://www.hhs.gov/ocr/hipaa

Gumby, S. S. (2008). Legal issues in teaching nursing. In B. K. Penn (Ed.), *Mastering the teaching role: A guide for nurse educators* (Chapter 3). Philadelphia, PA: F.A. Davis Company.

National Council of State Boards of Nursing. (n.d.). Purpose. Retrieved January 18, 2010, from www.ncsbn.org

Nelson, M. J. (2003). Ethical, legal, and economic foundations of the educational process. In S. B. Bastable (Ed.), *Nurse as educator: Principles of teaching and learning for nursing practice* (2nd ed.). Sudbury, MA: Jones and Bartlett Publishers.

O'Connor, K. F. (2010). Teaching nursing ethics. In L. Caputi (Ed.), *Teaching nursing: The art and science* (2nd ed., Vol. I). Glen Ellyn, IL: College of DuPage Press.

Rainbow, C. (2002). Descriptions of ethical theories and principles. Retrieved February 12, 2010, from http://www.bio.davidson.edu/people/kabernd/indep/carainbow/Theories.htm

Sumner, J. (2011). Ethics and nursing research. In C. Boswell & S. Cannon (Eds.), *Introduction to nursing research: Incorporating evidence-based practice* (2nd ed., pp. 55–91). Sudbury, MA: Jones and Bartlett Publishers.

Tippitt, M. P., Ard, N., Kline, J. R., Tilghman, J., Chamberlain, B., & Meagher, G. P. (2009). Creating environments that foster academic integrity. *Nursing Education Perspective*, 30(4), 239–244.

Web Links

The Family Educational Rights and Privacy Act (FERPA) is available at www.edu.gov/policy/gen/guide/fpco/ferpa/index.html.

The Health Insurance Portability and Accountability Act (HIPAA) is available at www.hhs.gov/ocr/hipaa.

The National Council of State Boards of Nursing purpose statement is available at www.ncsbn.org.

The American Nurses Association *Code of Ethics for Nurses with Interpretive Statements* is available at www.nursingworld.org/ethics/code/protected-nwcde813.htm.

The International Council of Nurses Code of Ethics for Nursing is available at www.icn.ch/icncode.pdf.

Multiple Choice Questions

1. The role of nursing faculty includes
   A. **ethical and legal implications in teaching nursing as well as the practice of nursing**.
   B. ethical and legal implications only in nursing practice.
   C. ethical and legal implications only in teaching nursing.
   D. none of the above.

   Rationale:

   Ethical and legal implications for teaching nursing require a balance of two perspectives, that of a practicing nurse and a nurse educator.

2. Ethics and laws are based on
   A. individual behaviors.
   B. opinions of the public.
   C. **the norms for societal behavior**.
   D. the values of family and friends.

   Rationale:

   The term *ethics* stems from the Greek word *ethos* and reflects standards. Laws are the norms for standards of societal behavior.

3. State Boards of Nursing protect
   A. students.
   B. faculty.
   C. administration.
   D. **the public**.

   Rationale:

   The purpose of state Boards of Nursing is to protect the welfare of the public and approve schools of nursing programs.

4. The Health Insurance Portability and Accountability Act (HIPAA) established standards about the use and disclosure of
   A. student information.
   B. faculty information.
   C. financial information.
   D. **health information**.

   Rationale:

   The Health Insurance Portability and Accountability Act (HIPAA) was enacted in 1996 to protect health information through a Privacy Rule to establish standards about the use and disclosure of health information.

5. For faculty members, HIPAA has
   A. no impact on their teaching role.
   B. major impact on their teaching role.
   C. implications for only hospitals/clinic staff.
   D. no implications for either the teaching or practice role.

Rationale:

HIPAA has a major impact on the role of nursing faculty members to ensure confidentiality of patient information on student clinical assignments, case study presentations, pre/postclinical conferences, student papers, and simulation lab scenarios.

6. The Family Educational Rights and Privacy Act (FERPA) protects
   A. parents.
   B. faculty.
   C. students.
   D. patients.

Rationale:

FERPA protects the privacy of student education records. After the age of 18, the right of access to the records transfers from the parents to the student.

7. FERPA applies to
   A. students, students with disabilities, and patients.
   B. parents, patients, and faculty.
   C. hospitals, clinics, and health departments.
   D. kindergarten, elementary, and high school students.

Rationale:

FERPA applies to students at all levels, students with disabilities, and students in clinical practice.

8. Regulatory agencies for health care, nursing, and nursing education set standards that apply to:
   A. the entertainment industry, television, and newspapers.
   B. higher education, hospital/clinics, and consumers of health care.
   C. all people in all countries for protection of endangered species.
   D. engineers, social workers, respiratory therapies, and nutritionists.

Rationale:

Regulatory agencies for health care, nursing, and nursing education set standards for higher education, hospitals/clinics, and consumers of health care. The legislative/regulatory agencies' standards are integral to the role of the nursing faculty.

9. When ethics and ethical principles are used effectively, decisions are based upon:

 A. **specific guidelines and information**.
 B. general protocols and data.
 C. specific guidelines and general data collected.
 D. general protocols and information.

Rationale:

When ethics is used effectively, decisions are based upon specific guidelines and information. The different ethical theories and principles provide the societal standards on which decisions can be made. O'Connor (2010) states that "learning to acknowledge personal moral views, to analyze and evaluate moral opinions, to reflect on moral situations, to defend moral choices, and to work with other healthcare team members on resolutions of ethical/moral situations and dilemmas is critical to the development of the ethical nurse" (p. 621).

10. The six major ethical principles are:

 A. trust, caring, autonomy, confidentiality, holism, and veracity.
 B. nonmalfeasance, caring, autonomy, confidentiality, veracity, and beneficence.
 C. **autonomy, veracity, nonmalfeasance, confidentiality, beneficence, and justice**.
 D. autonomy, trust, holism, nonmalfeasance, beneficence, and justice.

Rationale:

The principles subsumed within ethical decisions are not laws in and of themselves, but are the foundational components which guide the behaviors used when confronted by situations outside the control of laws. The six major ethical principles are: autonomy, veracity, nonmalfeasance, confidentiality, beneficence, and justice. Each of these tenets is used to maneuver toward an outcome when a situation is not covered by legal precedents.

11. The areas which help to shape an individual's unique decisions within the ethical dimension are:

 A. stress, justice, and emotions.
 B. motivation, work experiences, and emotions.
 C. **motivation, emotions, and life experiences**.
 D. life experiences, work experiences, and emotions.

Rationale:

Rainbow (2002) states that "each man deserves respect because only he has had those exact life experiences and understands his emotions, motivations, and body in such an intimate manner" (para. 5). These emotions, motivations, and life experiences shape how an individual comes to the unique decisions encountered in the ethical dimension. Within the principle of autonomy, each individual is allowed to pull from his or her culture and environment when making those decisions which are not addressed by legal rules.

12. Several different ethical theories are available to be used for the determination of an ethical decision. The theories are:
   A. deontological, utilitarianism, teleological, and consequentialism.
   B. virtual, care, and rights.
   C. deontological, virtual, care, and rights.
   D. deontology, consequentialism, virtue, care, and rights.

Rationale:

Several different theories are currently embraced—deontology, utilitarianism (consequentialist or teleological), virtue ethics, care ethics, and rights ethics. Each of these theories considers the ethical situation from a different approach, thus resulting in discrete management of the state of affairs.

13. Within the teaching realm, ethical decision making frequently addresses:
   A. the management of individuals instead of their physical care.
   B. the physical care of individuals instead of their management.
   C. both the physical and the individual component.
   D. neither the physical nor the individual component.

Rationale:

The nurse at the bedside deals with ethical situations which tend to relate to the physical side of professional practice. Life, death, quality of life, quantity of life, informed consent, privacy/confidentiality, and other aspects tend to be the focus for ethical situations which tend to impact the physical care of the client. Ethics within the teaching realm moves toward the management of individuals. Usually within the teaching realm, faculty members do not worry about whether their students are going to live or die. It is more about the moral development of the individual instead of the physical management of the individual.

14. An example of demonstrating ethical behavior by a faculty member would be
   A. assigning seats for the students within the classroom setting.
   B. restricting the objects a student can bring into a testing area.
   C. using student discussion groups to struggle with an ethical dilemma.
   D. telling students that they do not need to be concerned with values clarification.

Rationale:

Some examples showcasing ethical behavior are: (1) acting as an ethical role model as decisions are made, (2) using student discussion groups to struggle with ethical dilemmas, (3) facilitating values-clarification activities to allow students to safely investigate their values, and (4) providing case studies that incorporate ethical principles in the management of the scenario.

15. What documents can be used as an underpinning for ethical discussions?

A. Medical journals, articles, and lawyer briefs
B. Nursing research articles
C. HIPPA and FERPA documents
D. ANA Code of Ethics and ICN Code of Ethics

Rationale:

The American Nurses Association (ANA) in 2001 revised and updated *The Code for Nurses with Interpretive Statements*. This document provides a universal foundation used by American nurses as they work within an ethical framework. Though we do not at this time have a unique code for nurse educators, the ethical principles maintained within the ANA code provide an underpinning which is acceptable in practice and educational settings. The ICN Code of Ethics is an international code provided for the global provision of nursing care.

16. When considering strategies related to ethical academic integrity, faculty members should

A. identify positive methods for ensuring that students maintain academic integrity.
B. institute any measure that will prevent students from employing unethical behaviors.
C. expect students to use whatever means that they can to be successful.
D. set students up for problems early in the course to demonstrate that academic misconduct will not be tolerated.

Rationale:

As faculty members strive to apply the ideas of ethical decision making and academic integrity to the educational setting, several strategies can be employed to diminish or avert academic misconduct, such as assigning seats for students, jumbling up the order of the test questions, restricting the things students are allowed to have available during an exam, and having all examinations proctored. Though these strategies are effective in reducing the potential for academic misconduct, they are frequently viewed as negative in nature. These strategies seek to prevent students from doing the problematic behavior, which implies that faculty members expect students to engage in academic misconduct. Using strategies that showcase the expectation that students should not participate in academic misconduct sets up a positive and supportive environment for learning.

Discussion Questions

1. How does your school of nursing address HIPAA and FERPA guidelines and standards?

Considerations:

Examine the two federal acts. Review your school's policies and procedures for confidentiality of students and patients. Ask questions of yourself about how you use both HIPAA and FERPA in your role as a nurse educator.

2. Apply the ethical principles of autonomy, veracity, nonmalfeasance, confidentiality, beneficence, and justice to the following scenario:

You are a novice nursing educator who is confronted by a group of students who have worked together to complete an assignment which was expected to be done as individual work. The syllabus does not clearly state that the assignment was to be individual work. From the instructions provided within the syllabus, it could be interpreted to allow for working as a group. The students did not clarify the assignment but just assumed that group work was allowed.

Considerations:

■ The six major ethical principles are autonomy, veracity, nonmalfeasance, confidentiality, beneficence, and justice. Each of these tenets is used to maneuver toward an outcome when a situation is not covered by legal precedents.

■ According to Nelson (2003), autonomy is related to the idea that each of us has the right to self-determine the aspects within our lives. Laws have been established to protect the ability of individuals to make decisions independently about situations encountered. Each person is understood to have the right and responsibly to make free choices about the decisions that are key to their private lives.

■ Veracity is understood to represent truth telling. In each decision that a person confronts, the expectation is that truthful information will be provided by all involved parties so that the affected individual can use the entirety of the information to make the appropriate decision.

■ The concept of nonmalfeasance basically means "do no harm." Within health care particularly, the idea of doing no harm to individuals is paramount. This principle of not harming someone is foundational within ethical aspects and is vital in the foundation of legal determination.

■ Confidentiality is viewed as the securing of all privileged information which is obtained as a result of professional capacity with a patient or client. In each and every situation, the maintaining of private information in a secure and protected manner is viewed as the standard.

■ The concept of beneficence is viewed as "doing good." For each and every situation, the focus is on making a decision that will lead to the best outcome for the greatest number of individuals involved.

■ Justice is viewed as the fairness of the situation. This concept strives to ensure equality for all individuals in regard to goods, services, and protection.

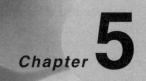

Connection Between Evidence-Based Practice and Nursing Education

Carol Boswell and Sharon Cannon

Chapter Objectives

At the conclusion of this chapter, the learner will be able to:

1. Recognize the key definitions and elements related to evidence-based practice and evidence-based teaching.
2. Analyze the different evidence-based practice theories/models to see how they apply to evidence-based teaching.
3. Discuss motivation of learners in nursing education.
4. Identify steps to foster motivation in students.
5. Compare compliance in nursing education to patient education.
6. Persuade students to maintain healthy behaviors.

Key Terms

➤ ACESTAR model

➤ ARCC model

➤ Cochrane Collaboration

➤ Compliance

➤ Health behavior

➤ Iowa model

➤ Joanna Briggs Institute

➤ Johns Hopkins model

➤ Model

➤ Motivation

➤ Rosswurn-Larrabee model

➤ Stetler/Marran model

➤ Theory

Introduction

At this point, the literature does not provide any theory or model for evidence-based teaching (EBT). Since there does not exist a theory/model for EBT, the models and theories provided for evidence-based practice (EBP) must be used to contribute key aspects. As the different EBP theories and models are considered, key elements within those resources can be pulled together to address the process of EBT. The application of the elements and concepts requires manipulation to address the academic and educational aspects of EBT. Most of the different pieces can be readily applied with a change in focus from a clinical to an educational concentration.

Benner, Sutphen, Leonard, and Day (2009) advocated for a radical transformation within the educating of nurses. Benner et al. (2009) argue that despite the substantial external challenges facing health care, nursing practice, and nursing education, changes within nursing education are imperative and essential. Within this text, the authors demand that nursing education deliberate and undertake a drastic and revolutionary change in the manner of delivery for nursing education. Some of the changes demanded by this call reflect the necessity of embracing EBT. The recommendations for nursing programs include changing:

■ from a focus on covering decontextualized knowledge to an emphasis on teaching for a sense of salience, situated cognition, and action in particular situations.
■ from a sharp separation of clinical and classroom teaching to an integration of the two.
■ from an emphasis on critical thinking to an emphasis on clinical reasoning and multiple ways of thinking.
■ from an emphasis on socialization and role taking to an emphasis on formation. (Benner et al., 2009, p. 4).

Each of these recommendations strongly supports the idea that the educational process used within the classroom and clinical settings must assimilate the process of confirming the appropriateness and effectiveness of the different teaching strategies utilized. To simply teach as we have always taught or been taught does not demonstrate the commitment to excellence which is mandated by this call for an uncompromising transformation in the educating of nursing professionals.

Definitions and Elements

As thoughts turn toward EBT, many different words come to mind that play a part in understanding the facets involved. Terms such as *theory, model, philosophy, nursing process, critical thinking, evidence-based practice, research, practice-based evidence,* and *research utilization* will be discussed. Though these terms are sometimes used interchangeably, each term provides a different dimension in the management of evidence. *Encarta World English Dictionary* (2009) defines *philosophy* as an investigation into the foundational concepts, a discipline of thought, the foundational or fundamental principles, and/or a compilation of beliefs and goals. The philosophical aspects are those items which come together to form the foundation on which the other building blocks can be laid upon. As one moves from the philosophy, theories are developed. *Encarta World English Dictionary* (2009) characterizes a **theory** as a set of rules and/or techniques that can be applied to a subject and/or abstract thoughts, the ideas that form the underpinning that is used to move a distinct practice into reality. Theories come in multiple levels and formations. Theories can be very structured and clearly delineated, or they can be the initial work toward understanding the abstract thoughts and ideas about a particular subject.

According to *Encarta World English Dictionary* (2009), a **model** is a simplified version of the complex analysis and problem solving related to a topic and/or an explanation of a theory and/or the concepts related to that theory. The model is usually an illustration of the complex fact, beliefs, rules, and thoughts that are subsumed within a theory. The model provides an attempt to visually represent the diverse interconnectedness of the concepts within a theory. Complexity theory is an example that demonstrates diversity through informal networking that involves interlocking relationships. The model for complexity theory includes patient care beyond the hospital setting and provides a microsystem approach to the level of care for populations of individuals, families, and population groups (Roussel, Godfrey, & Williams, 2010). Models provide the foundation for the manner in which relationships are formed and managed.

Within EBP, many different terms come into play. As is true with any involvement with evidence, thought and analysis are key. Terms such as *nursing process, critical thinking, research,* and *research utilization* all depict some form of thinking and scrutinizing. The nursing process includes assessment, diagnosis, planning, implementation, and evaluation. Each of these different steps comes together to move a patient treatment plan forward toward success. These same five steps are critical for the provision of appropriate and effective nursing education. The nursing process provides a foundation for the effective management of EBT. A second term which is directly involved in analysis is *critical* thinking. According to The Critical Thinking Co. (2005), "critical thinking is the identification and evaluation of evidence to guide decision making. A critical thinker uses broad in-depth analysis of evidence to make decisions and communicate his/her beliefs clearly and accurately" (para. 1). The concepts included in thinking critically require that each problem and/or topic is considered from all sides. Each and every potential aspect housed within critical thinking compels the participants to seek innovative ways to address the various components in an evaluation of the evidence. Critical thinking, though imperative for nursing care, is also vital to the process of educating the student. It is important that faculty members model the process of critical thinking in the classroom and clinical setting, use it when making decisions about management of the classroom, and employ it with each and every discussion during the educational process.

Other terms frequently included during a discussion of EBP are *research* and *research utilization*. Research is defined as the systematic examination of a topic to ascertain facts, to determine or modify a theory/model, or to cultivate a plan of action established on the evidence revealed (*Encarta World English Dictionary*, 2009). Research utilization builds on the idea of research. Research utilization considers the evidence presented as a result of one study. When multiple research projects are summarized, the outcome includes a systematic review.

The final terms to consider are *evidence-based practice, practice-based evidence*, and *evidence-based teaching*. These terms were carefully contemplated within Chapter 1. A comparison of the different definitions for EBP was provided in Table 1-1. Six different definitions were contrasted. The characteristics within each of the definitions were provided to determine the consistency among the definitions. According to Boswell and Cannon (2011), the constant characteristics found within the multiple definitions relate to the decision-making scheme, clinical application, provider expertise, and client contribution. According to Drisko (2008b), "EBP is a mix of a) learning what treatments 'work' based on the best available research (whether experiential or not), b) discussing client views about the treatment to consider cultural and other differences, and to honor client self determination and autonomy, c) considering the professional's 'clinical wisdom' based on work with similar and dissimilar cases that may provide a context for understanding the research evidence, and d) considering what the professional can, and can not, provide fully and ethically" (para. 2). Each of these four components is critical to the provision of EBP. The evidence, client, setting, and provider are all crucial as effective and appropriate care is considered and determined. We would suggest that while research evidence is tested and analyzed, other evidence is also appropriate to consider when determining the best practices to be implemented. As we move EBP to practice-based evidence, the process takes on a convoluted appearance. EBP is viewed as the general level of identifying and validating the evidence presented and related to the different topics under investigation. Practice-based evidence takes the evidence as it moves from the "research to practice" level. Thus, practice-based evidence is the day-to-day engagement of the evidence into the practice arena for the betterment of the provision of care.

One last term to consider for this discussion is *evidence-based teaching*. As was stated in Chapter 1, EBT is a dynamic, holistic system using educational principles validated by evidence to support, maintain, and promote a new level of knowledge for a learner in a variety of settings. Drisko (2008a) suggested that "educational efforts . . . could be oriented to provide beginning professionals with effective tools and a model for the continuing improvement and renewal of their professional practices" (para. 1). EBT takes the ideas and concepts included within EBP to gain an improved management of the educational process within the health disciplines. Chapter 1 provided several figures and discussion concerning the process of EBT for use within this text.

Theory/Models

Many different types of EBP theories and models exist. According to Vratny and Shriver (2007), EBP models concentrate on the scientific nature, not the "art," of EBP. Nursing knowledge tends to emerge from clinical experiences, human sources, opinion, folklore, rituals, and/ or traditions, but not usually from research. It seems that up to this point in the nursing profession, the knowledge used by nurses has been based on these aspects. As a result of these knowledge sources, the boundaries between research, research utilization, and EBP have been clouded. Only in the last few years has the nursing profession embraced the concept of EBP. With this transition to evidence as the foundation for the care provided by nurses, nursing research has increased. In addition, discussions have multiplied and focused on areas concerning: What is evidence? Where can evidence be found? How much evidence is needed? What about the "art" of nursing care as a source for this evidence? While some progress toward the answers to these questions has been made, additional attention and thought are needed.

Since multiple models and theories about EBP have been developed, Gawlinski and Rutledge (2008) provided an evaluation tool for critiquing the different EBP models. This tool provides an initial method for selecting a model that could be utilized in the unique practices of nursing care. Each setting has to carefully consider the different models and theories to select one that works best within the unique environment. This tool is one method developed to facilitate the selection of a model that would address the concerns and problems distinctive to a given setting.

At this point, we need to look at several of the EBP models. While these models are EBP models, they have aspects which can be related to EBT. Since no EBT models exist at this time, the application of EBP models is the primary method for viewing the process. Two overarching groups—Joanne Briggs Institute and the Cochrane Collaboration—will be discussed first. These two agencies do not directly have models but are strategic when looking at EBP. After discussing these two agencies, several EBP models will be presented: Stetlers/Marran, Rosswurn-Larrabee, ACESTAR, ARCC, Iowa, and Johns Hopkins. Theses are not the only models but tend to be the ones that are frequently utilized.

The **Joanna Briggs Institute** (JBI) was established in 1996. Evidence-based health care is regarded as a cyclical opportunity by the members of this institution. The JBI strives to incorporate all levels of evidence from opinion up to the rigorous random controlled trials (RCTs) while endeavoring to focus on the effectiveness of interventions and activities. In order to ensure that the information and resources provided by JBI are of global importance, they:

- Consider international evidence related to the feasibility, appropriateness, meaningfulness, and effectiveness of healthcare interventions (evidence generation).
- Include these different forms of evidence in a formal assessment called a systematic review (evidence synthesis).
- Globally disseminate information in appropriate, relevant formats to inform health systems, health professionals, and consumers (evidence transfer).
- Offer designated programs to enable the effective implementation of evidence and evaluation of its impact on healthcare practice (evidence utilization). (JBI, 2008)

The JBI uses as its primary crux feasibility, appropriateness, meaningfulness, and effectiveness of health practices and delivery methods (JBI, 2008). These four principal designations make up the "FAME" scale of evidence. In addition to the JBI Levels of Evidence scale, the JBI also utilizes a JBI Grading of Recommendation scale that also uses the four designations. These two scales mirror the Appraisal of Guidelines Research and Evaluation (AGREE) Collaboration.

The **Cochrane Collaboration** is an international, not-for-profit network established in 1993 to help healthcare providers and others to make well-informed healthcare decisions. This collaboration was named after Archie Cochrane, a British epidemiologist, who is viewed as the individual who conceptualized EBP (Cochrane Collaboration, n.d.). This group pledges to keep up-to-date and accurate information about health care and its effects for the global community. One of the major contributions from this agency is the production and dissemination of systematic reviews concerning healthcare interventions. It also is dedicated to promoting the ongoing search for evidence in the form of clinical trials and other studies of intervention. Those who generate the reviews are primarily volunteer healthcare professionals who function in one of the many Cochrane Review Groups. These groups work with an editorial team to prepare and maintain the reviews while applying the rigorous quality standards for which Cochrane Reviews are known. The Cochrane Reviews are viewed as the gold standard in regard to the process and quality of the publications.

The **Stetler/Marran model** of research utilization was developed in 1976, making it one of the oldest of the models. It was revised in 1994 with the addition of conceptual underpinnings and a set of assumptions, and is now referred to as the Stetler model. According to Gawlinski and Rutledge (2008), this model is one of the few that does not pivot on only formal changes accomplished by nurses within the organizational setting. This model assimilates the individual nurse while promoting the use of both internal and external data/evidence. According to Melnyk and Fineout-Overholt (2005), "the Stetler model outlines a prescriptive series of steps to assess and use research findings, thereby facilitating safe and effective EBP" (p. 188). The Stetler model is a practitioner-oriented model that focuses on critical thinking and the incorporation of the findings of knowledgeable individuals. The steps included within the model are:

- Preparation (ascertaining the rationale and core of the review)
- Validation (confirming the research as to applicability and relevancy)
- Comparative evaluation (reviewing findings from comparable studies)
- Decision making (selecting from four choices—to use the findings, to consider using the findings, to delay using the findings, or to reject the findings in total)
- Translation/application (determining how to implement the findings into practice)
- Evaluation (validating the consequence on the practice, policy, and/or patient) (McClinton, 1997)

Overall, the changes to this model have been accomplished to address the utilization of focused integrative review methodology, targeted evidence concepts, and ongoing encounters as the model has been used by clinical nurse specialists and nurse practitioners. Although this model is not a true EBP model, it serves as the forerunner to the models which have been developed as a result of moving from research utilization toward practice based on sound evidence.

The **Rosswurn–Larrabee model** was developed in 1999. This model was established for use in primary care settings with advanced practitioners. It strives to guide the individual through the entire process of EBP. The steps used within this model follow the steps of the nursing process. The six steps are: assessing the needs of stakeholders, building bridges while making connections, synthesizing the evidence to determine its relevancy, planning the practice change, implementing the changes culminating in evaluating those changes, and integrating the practice changes for sustainability. This model aspired to move the existing medical EBP model to include a focus on nursing phenomena. The ultimate goal within this model is to change clinical practice as a result of the evidence. According to Gawlinski and Rutledge (2008), the preliminary need for change was ascertained by equating the internal data with data resulting from studies conducted outside of the organization. Thus, the internal data were supported by the external information that was collected and analyzed.

Another model was developed by the Academic Center for Evidence-based Practice (ACEP). The model is entitled the ACE Star Model of Knowledge Transformation, or the **ACESTAR model**. According to the ACEP (2005), "the Star Model of Knowledge Transformation is a model for understanding the cycles, nature, and characteristics of knowledge that are utilized in various aspects of evidence-based practice" (p. 1). The model is depicted as a star with the five points embracing: knowledge discovery, evidence summary, translation into practice recommendations, integration into practice, and evaluation. According to Gawlinski and Rutledge (2008), this model supports EBP by depicting knowledge as it evolves. This model does not discuss the use of nonresearch evidence. Knowledge gained from other venues outside of research is not integrated within the model. Although the model does not completely restrict the incorporation of knowledge gained in this manner, the assimilation of other knowledge is done by the individual, not within the explanation of the stages.

The Advancing Research and Clinical Practice Through Close Collaboration model, or **ARCC model**, has as its goals: (1) the advancement of EBP among advanced practice nurses, (2) the establishment of a network of clinicians to act as EBP mentors, and (3) dissemination of the best evidence. Initially, this model focused on RCTs. As it has matured, other levels of evidence have been accepted but the focus continues to be directed toward research findings. Gawlinski and Rutledge (2008) designate the key focus for this model to be at the departmental and/or unit level within the organization. The ARCC draws on the use of EBP mentors to champion the development of the advanced practice nurse. This model endeavors to consolidate the integration of practice and research in the form of EBP with a foundation of benchmarking.

The Iowa Model of Evidence-Based Practice to Promote Quality Care, or the **Iowa model**, was originally developed in 1994 with a goal of using it to guide bedside nursing staff members toward the use of research findings to improve the care provided. This model emphasizes the organization, primarily acute care settings. Melnyk and Fineout-Overholt (2005) stated that the utilization of this model "gives a strong message to the organization about its role in the support of EBP" (p. 197). The Iowa model was cultivated to promote quality care in multiple academic and clinical settings. It works to mesh quality improvement with research utilization. One item unique to this model is the use of "triggers" of EBP. The triggers are those items identified within the practice arena that raise a question as to the validity of the current practice. By identifying and acknowledging these triggers, EBP projects can be instituted to determine the optimum way to address the issue that will result in quality care for clients.

The final EBP model to be discussed within this chapter is the **Johns Hopkins model**. According to Johns Hopkins Nursing and Evidence-Based Practice (n.d.), this model "is a powerful problem-solving approach to clinical decision-making and is accompanied by user-friendly tools to guide individual or group use" (para. 1). This model was developed for use by the nurses and nursing students at Johns Hopkins to answer clinical, administrative, and education practice questions.

While multiple EBP models and tools are available, their application to teaching has not occurred at this time. Each of these models has concepts that could be adapted to address the EBT viewpoint. Figure 1-2 reflects the multiple areas which must be considered when conceptualizing the aspects indicative of EBT. The facets and features encompassed by the teaching role are multiple and complex. Care must be given to ensure that while the academic teaching role is a huge component of the educational process, other educational venues such as staff development are also of paramount importance. As evidence is collected on the different facets and features included in the teaching role, the application of the evidence needs to embrace the multiplexity of the teaching role and environment.

Motivation, Compliance, and Health Behaviors of the Learner

Having examined EBP theories, models, definitions, and elements, and understanding of the **motivation** of students is essential. Reams of evidence regarding motivation abound in the literature, especially in the behavioral science and education areas. Theories of motivation are provided by Skinner, Piaget, Bandura, Maslow, and Knowles, to name just a few. However, few studies have been conducted in nursing education. An examination of motivational theories will be discussed first.

Ard (2009) suggests that motivation may look simple but is actually complex; Ard applies Wlodkowaki's 1978 definition of motivation as involving processes promoting and directing the purpose of behavior. Ard (2009) builds on that definition by indicating that "motivation is a complex interaction" (p. 41) that is both intrinsic (within) and extrinsic (external). However, Biehler and Snowman suggest "motivation is only intrinsic but circumstances can be created to influence motivation" ("Motivation," 1997, p. 2).

We are all familiar with Skinner's model of operant conditioning that involved rats in a maze seeking a piece of cheese. Skinner indicates that positive or negative reinforcement determines motivation ("Motivation," 1997). Ever wonder what Skinner might have thought about "Who moved my cheese"? Within this book about managing change, the use of positive and/or negative reinforcement can help greatly as change is addressed. The use of reinforcements to drive the conditioning is a key strategy incorporated into Skinner's model.

Piaget took a more cognitive approach to motivation by explaining it as a balance between old and new experiences using organizing and balancing schemes. As a result, learners want to "master their environment" ("Motivation," 1997, p. 3).

Sweetland (2010) defines motivation as "the force that drives a person to do something" (p. 1). He further emphasizes that motivation comes from within the individual, which Bandura identifies as goal setting and modification of prior behavior models that are successful. Hodson-Carlton (2009) also points out the importance of Bandura's theory related to self-efficacy, which "is the result of previous learning attempts." (p. 312).

According to Biehler and Snowman ("Motivation," 1997), Maslow's hierarchy of needs ranges from a deficiency of needs to a growth need (self-actualization) to achieve self-fulfillment. Cognitive needs for growth influence motivation.

In higher education, Malcolm Knowles's theory of adult learning is considered essential to motivating students. Knowles proposes that adults are self-directed, need to be involved, rely on prior experiences, need relevance, and should center on problems rather than content [Andragogy, (M. Knowles), 2010)]. In many ways, one could postulate that Knowles's theory incorporates all of the motivational theories previously discussed.

For the purpose of this text, motivation is considered to be both intrinsic and extrinsic. Motivation involves satisfaction derived from prior learning prompting the desire to learn more.

Now let's investigate evidence regarding motivation of students in nursing education. Ard (2009) suggests that a "literature review revealed only five studies on motivation in nursing" (p. 4) and all were conducted outside of the United States. Thompson (2009) supports Ard's suggestion that there is a lack of nursing education research and little evidence to validate learning theories. Most of the motivational literature in nursing education is descriptive applications or strategies that provide nurse educators information about motivation. Research about what motivates student nurses and how nurse educators influence motivation of students are two areas worthy of intense study.

Inherent to education, patient education, or nursing education is the notion of compliance. **Compliance** is discussed in almost every aspect of the management of health care, especially in relation to patient education. You can often hear comments such as, "I gave them the information but they don't use it," or "I taught it, so why don't they incorporate the knowledge?" Obviously, compliance is closely related to motivation (i.e., the impetus to move/change/act). Getting patients or nursing students to change behavior and act on information given is a phenomenal task and may overwhelm novice or even expert nurse educators. Though little research has been conducted in this area, it does not mean that there aren't strategies to increase compliance and motivation.

Based on the motivational theories discussed previously, tips proposed by the authors will be examined. One of the first tips to consider in motivation of learners is the differences among the generations of learners, as discussed in Chapter 2. Patient education has focused more heavily on adult learning and literacy, especially health literacy. However, nursing education has recognized the importance of generational differences. Use of these generational considerations are discussed in throughout this book, as it is an important aspect to incorporate into motivating students to learn.

ARCS-motivation theory (Keller, 2010) suggests that to motivate, the educator must address attention, relevance, confidence, and satisfaction (ARCS). Attention can be achieved through novel and uncertain events, through posing problems, and through variations of instructional elements. Relevance relates to familiar language and examples, goals to be accomplished, and matching teaching strategies with profiles of students. Confidence is gained when learners know how to perform at multiple achievement levels and are given supportive feedback. Satisfaction involves opportunities to use knowledge in real or simulated settings, provision of positive feedback and reinforcement, and use of consistent standards and consequences to accomplish tasks.

Knowles (2010) focuses heavily on relevance of task-orientation, discovery, experimentation, involvement in the instructions, and problem-oriented content. Process is emphasized more than content being taught, with faculty more in the role of facilitator than lecturer.

In motivation theory, Sweetland (2010) offers 14 suggestions to increase motivation. The suggestions include discussion about variables (ability, luck, efforts, etc.), positive feedback on progress, opportunities to create knowledge, relearning concepts and correcting errors, listening and teaching how to listen, maintaining high expectations, and problem solving with critical thinking.

Biehler and Snowman ("Motivation," 1997) suggest the use of behavioral techniques, addressing what is required with the process and achievement, satisfying deficiency needs, emphasizing rewards and consequences, focusing on success, and having a sense of adventure. They incorporate both operant conditioning and social learning theory.

Also, tips and strategies will be given in additional chapters for online, clinical, and simulation settings.

As we strive to integrate generational components and motivational theories, care must be given to the use of generalizations. Generalizations must be considered with the awareness that each individual is unique. Utilizing the information provided in Chapter 2 regarding generational characteristics, some assumptions related to motivation can be ascertained.

The Veterans (born before 1945) tend to reflect the concepts found within the ARCS-motivation theory. This generation strives to serve while working hard and respecting authority. To motivate students within this cohort, attention should be given to clearly: (1) determine the goals or tasks expected; (2) embrace the attributes of discipline, order, structure, and logic; and (3) address the idea of duty.

Moving to the Baby Boomer cohort (born 1946–1964), the mechanisms to consider would center on this generation needing to be in the spotlight. While embracing the idea of "making a difference," they tend to be focused on themselves—the "Me" generation. Members of this generation, though team players, desire personal gratification. As faculty members attempt to challenge and motivate these individuals, thoughts should be directed toward providing recognition for activities completed. The Baby Boomer cohort embraces challenges and risks. They function well when allowed to discover answers, experiment with options, and problem solve, particularly within groups.

The next cohort for consideration is Generation X (born 1965–1976). When trying to motivate this group, it is wise to remember that they are self-starters and results-driven. Providing goals for them then getting out of their way to allow them to creatively and individually complete the goals is beneficial. This cohort expects to influence the terms and conditions employed to research the goals and outcomes.

The final group currently at the higher education level is the Millennial generation (born 1977–1997). This cohort tends to be very competitive, civic minded, and materialistic. When endeavoring to motivate this group, employing challenges based on "real-world" situations allows them the opportunity to compete with peers to solve an identifiable problem. The Millennial cohort is goal-driven. Motivation is increased as the goals are set and confronted within a team orientation.

The Veterans and Generation Xers want to work independently toward their goals. Baby Boomers and Millennial individuals value the benefits of teamwork to reach a goal/outcome. Another aspect to consider related to motivating the different generations concerns time orientation. Members of the Veteran and Baby Boomer groups are more structured concerning time; they are thus more linear. The other two cohorts (Generation X and Millennial) tend to be more "outside the box" due to their technology orientation. Technology allows these groups to work flexibly, any time and any place.

Although the generational characteristics are useful when considering motivation, care must be used to ensure that each individual is still considered in relation to personal needs and expectations. Faculty members need to contemplate the distinctive and idiosyncratic characteristics of each student and/or class cohort. Each class tends to take on a distinct group personality. The generational characteristics which are included in the class cohort can help the faculty member to have a beginning place from which to seek to engage and motivate the class.

Summary Thoughts

Evidence-based practice and evidence-based teaching share elements and concepts applicable to the advancement of nursing education. While research utilizing EBP elements and concepts is becoming more prolific, a dearth of research exists in nursing education. Evidence-based practice models can and should be applied to nursing education. Benner et al. (2009) advocate for drastic change in the delivery of nursing education. Evidence for promoting best practices in the classroom and clinical setting must incorporate the motivation and compliance of students to critically think when providing nursing care, especially to patients from diverse settings and having complex health-care needs.

Summary Points

1. Currently, the literature does not provide any theory or model for EBT.
2. The recommendations presented by the call for a radical change in nursing education strongly support the idea that the educational process used within classroom and clinical settings must assimilate the process of confirming the appropriateness and effectiveness of the different teaching strategies utilized.
3. EBT is a dynamic, holistic system using educational principles validated by evidence to support, maintain, and promote a new level of knowledge for a learner in a variety of settings.
4. Nursing knowledge tends to emerge from clinical experiences, human sources, opinion, folklore, rituals, and/or traditions, but not usually from research.
5. The Joanna Briggs Institute strives to incorporate all levels of evidence, from opinion up to the rigorous RCT, while endeavoring to focus on the effectiveness of interventions and activities.
6. The Joanna Briggs Institute uses as its primary crux feasibility, appropriateness, meaningfulness, and effectiveness (FAME) of health practices and delivery methods.
7. One of the major contributions from the Cochrane Collaboration is the production and dissemination of systematic reviews concerning health-care interventions.
8. As evidence is collected on the different facets and features included in the teaching role, the application of the evidence needs to embrace the multiplexity of the teaching role and environment.
9. Motivation is intrinsic and extrinsic.
10. Motivation appears simple but is complex.
11. Few studies have been conducted in the United States that involve the learning motivation of nursing students.
12. Consideration of generational characteristics can be effective when determining how to motivate a cohort of students.

Tips for Nurse Educators to Use

1. Develop a clear definition of EBP and EBT.
2. Incorporate an evidence-based model approach to EBT.
3. Consider generational differences when seeking to motivate students.
4. Promote attention, relevance, confidence, and satisfaction to engage students in the learning process.
5. Utilize feedback, listening, and problem solving/critical thinking.
6. Emphasize rewards, consequences, and success while maintaining high expectations.
7. Incorporate operant conditioning and social learning theory.

References

Academic Center for Evidence-Based Practice. (2005). ACE: Learn about EBP. Retrieved March 17, 2010, from http://acestar.uthscsa.edu/Learn_model.htm

Ard, N. (2009). Essentials of learning. In C. M. Schultz (Ed.), Building a science of nursing education: Foundation for evidence-based teaching-learning. (Chapter 3, pp. 25–131). New York, NY: National League for Nursing.

Benner, P., Sutphen, M., Leonard, V., & Day, L. (2009). Book highlights from educating nurses: A call for radical transformation. Hoboken, NJ: Jossey-Bass Publishers.

Boswell, C., & Cannon, S. (2011). Introduction to nursing research: Incorporating evidence-based practice (2nd ed.). Sudbury, MA: Jones and Bartlett Publishers.

Cochrane Collaboration. (n.d.). About us. Retrieved March 17, 2010, from www.cochrane.org/about-us

Drisko, J. (2008a). Evidence-based practice. Retrieved March 16, 2010, from http://sophia.smith.edu/~jdrisko/evidence_based_practice.htm

Drisko, J. (2008b). What is EBP? Retrieved March 16, 2010, from http://sophia.smith.edu/~jdrisko/what_is_ebp.htm

Encarta World English Dictionary [North American Edition]. (2009). Retrieved March 16, 2010, from www.bing.com/Dictionary

Gawlinski, A., & Rutledge, D. (2008). Selecting a model for evidence-based practice changes: A practical approach. AACN Advanced Critical Care, 19(3), 291–300.

Hodson-Carlton, K. E. (2009). The learning resource center. In C. M. Schultz, Building a science of nursing education: Foundation for evidence-based teaching-learning. (Chapter 18, pp. 303–321). New York, NY: National League for Nursing.

Joanna Briggs Institute. (2008). Joanna Briggs Institute model of evidence-based health care. Retrieved March 17, 2010, from www.joannabriggs.au

Johns Hopkins Nursing and Evidence-Based Practice. (n.d.). About the Johns Hopkins nursing EBP model. Retrieved March 17, 2010, from www.ijhn.edu/contEd_3rdLevel_Class.asp

Keller, J. (2010). ARCS-motivation theory. Retrieved February 8, 2010, from http://ide.ed.psu.edu/idde/ARCS.htm

Knowles, M. (n.d.). Andragogy. Retrieved February 28, 2010, from http://tips.psychology.org/Knowles.html

McClinton, J. (1997). Stetler model of research utilization. Retrieved March 17, 2010, from www.kumc.edu/instruction/nursing/NRSG754/SYLLABUS/stetlermodel.html

Melnyk, B. M., & Fineout-Overholt, E. (2005). Evidence-based practice in nursing & healthcare: A guide to best practice. Philadelphia, PA: Lippincott Williams & Wilkins.

Motivation. (1997). In R. Biehler & J. Snowman (Eds.), Psychology applied to teaching (Chapter 11, pp. 1–10). Boston, MA: Houghton Mifflin. Retrieved February 8, 2010, from http://www.college.cengage.com/education/pbl/tc/motivate.html

Roussel, L., Godfrey, A. J., & Williams, L. (2010). Community resources awareness and networking through advocacy. In J. L. Harris & L. Roussel (Eds.), Initiating and sustaining the clinical nurse leader role: A practical guide (Chapter 10, pp. 171–182). Sudbury, MA: Jones and Bartlett Publishers.

Sweetland, R. (2010). Motivational theory. Retrieved February 8, 2010, from www.homeofbob.com/cman/general/motivation/motivatn.html

The Critical Thinking Co. (2005). Critical thinking. Retrieved March 16, 2010, from www.criticalthinking.com/company/articles/critical-thinking-definition.jsp

Thompson, C. (2009). Teaching-learning in the cognitive domains. In C. M. Schultz (Ed.), *Building a science of nursing education: Foundation for evidence-based teaching-learning* (Chapter 4, pp. 133–176). New York, NY: National League for Nursing.

Vratny, A., & Shriver, D. (2007). A conceptual model for growing evidence-based practice. *Nursing Administration Quarterly, 31*(2), 162–170.

Web Links

View the Joanna Briggs Institute home page at www.joannabriggs.edu.au.
View the Cochrane Collaboration home page at www.cochrane.org.
The ACESTAR model is available at http://acestar.uthscsa.edu.
The Iowa model is available at www.uihealthcare.com/depts/nursing/rqom.
The Johns Hopkins model is available at www.jhspk.edu/epc.

Multiple Choice Questions

1. The nursing process that provides a beginning organization for thinking includes

A. **assessment, diagnosis, planning, implementation, and evaluation**.
B. assessment, data mining, implementation, and evaluation.
C. planning, organizing, diagnosis, implementation, and evaluation.
D. planning, diagnosis, data mining, implementation, and evaluation.

Rationale:

The nursing process includes the phases of assessment, diagnosis, planning, implementation, and evaluation. Each of these different steps comes together to move a patient treatment plan forward toward success.

2. The characteristics routinely found in the multiple evidence-based practice definitions are

A. decision making, educational application, and client contribution.
B. clinical application, physician expertise, and client contribution.
C. critical thinking, clinical application, and provider expertise.
D. **decision making, provider expertise, and clinical application**.

Rationale:

According to Boswell and Cannon (2011), the constant characteristics found within the multiple definitions are the decision-making scheme, clinical application, provider expertise, and client contribution.

3. Evidence-based teaching is a

A. complex process using educational principles legalized by data to aid the learner to gain knowledge.
B. **dynamic, holistic system using educational principles validated by evidence to support, maintain, and promote knowledge for a learner in a variety of settings**.
C. energetic system employing principles of education to provide knowledge to a learner in a variety of settings to support and maintain the process.
D. holistic system using educational principles validated by evidence to support, maintain, and promote a new level of knowledge for a learner in a classroom setting.

Rationale:

Evidence-based teaching is a dynamic, holistic system using educational principles validated by evidence to support, maintain, and promote a new level of knowledge for a learner in a variety of settings.

4. The Joanna Briggs Institute uses four principles and/or criteria when determining the scale of evidence, which are

A. assessment, planning, implementation, and evaluation.

B. feasibility, assessment, meaningfulness, and effectiveness.

C. feasibility, appropriateness, meaningfulness, and effectiveness.

D. assessment, appropriateness, meaningfulness, and evaluation.

Rationale:

The Joanna Briggs Institute uses as it primary crux feasibility, appropriateness, meaningfulness, and effectiveness of health practices and delivery methods (JBI, 2008). These four principal designations make up the "FAME" scale of evidence.

5. The two scales used by the Joanna Briggs Institute for assessing evidence mirror what other guide?

A. Appraisal of Guidelines Research and Evaluation (AGREE) Collaboration

B. FAME scale of evidence

C. Cochrane Collaboration

D. Appraisal Related to Competency and Completeness (ARCC)

Rationale:

In addition to the JBI Levels of Evidence scale, JBI also utilizes a JBI Grading of Recommendation scale that also uses the four designations. These two scales mirror the Appraisal of Guidelines Research and Evaluation (AGREE) Collaboration.

6. The gold standard in regard to the process and quality of systematic reviews is the

A. Joanna Briggs Institute.

B. Academic Center for Evidence-based Practice.

C. Institute of Medicine.

D. Cochrane Reviews.

Rationale:

One of the major contributions from the Cochrane Collaboration is the production and dissemination of systematic reviews concerning healthcare interventions. It also is dedicated to promoting the ongoing search for evidence in the form of clinical trials and other studies of intervention. Those who generate the reviews are primarily volunteer healthcare professionals who function in one of the many Cochrane Review Groups. These groups work with an editorial team to prepare and maintain the reviews while applying the rigorous quality standards for which Cochrane Reviews are known. The Cochrane Reviews are viewed as the gold standard in regard to the process and quality of the publications.

7. The model that serves as the forerunner for evidence-based practice models is the

   A. Rosswurn-Larrabee model.
   B. ACESTAR model.
   C. Stetler model.
   D. ARCC model.

Rationale:

Overall, the changes to the Stetler model have been accomplished to address the utilization of focused integrative review methodology, targeted evidence concepts, and ongoing encounters as the model has been used by clinical nurse specialists and nurse practitioners. Although this model is not a true EBP model, it serves as the forerunner to the models that have been developed as a result of moving from research utilization toward practice based upon sound evidence.

8. The evidence-based practice model that focuses on knowledge is the

   A. Rosswurn-Larrabee model.
   B. ACESTAR model.
   C. Stetler model.
   D. ARCC model.

Rationale:

The ACESTAR model, according to the Academic Center for Evidence-based Practice (2005), "is a model for understanding the cycles, nature, and characteristics of knowledge that are utilized in various aspects of evidence-based practice" (p. 1).

9. Motivation is

   A. intrinsic.
   B. extrinsic.
   C. both intrinsic and extrinsic.
   D. neither intrinsic nor extrinsic.

Rationale:

Motivational theories postulate that motivation is both intrinsic and extrinsic.

10. Motivation involves processes that

   A. look simple but are complex.
   B. conflict with established research.
   C. have little relevance to teaching.
   D. apply only to the science of psychology.

Rationale:

Ard (2009) suggests that motivation may look simple but is actually complex.

11. Validation of learning is

    A. found in empirical studies in nursing education.

    B. seldom discussed in descriptive applications.

    C. not necessary to be an effective nurse educator.

    D. found in only five studies, all of which were conducted outside of the United States.

Rationale:

Ard (2009) notes that a "literature review revealed only five studies on motivation in nursing" (p. 4), and all were conducted outside of the United States.

12. Changing behavior and acting on information given are two aspects to consider for

    A. self-confidence.

    B. apathy.

    C. indifference.

    D. motivation.

Rationale:

Compliance is closely related to motivation (i.e. the impetus to move/act/change).

13. According to Keller, the ARCS-motivation theory must address

    A. attention, relevance, confidence, and satisfaction.

    B. activity, response, caring, and satisfaction.

    C. attention, response, commonalities, and satisfaction.

    D. activity, response, complexity, and sources.

Rationale:

Keller's (2010) ARCS-motivation theory suggests that to motivate learners, the educator must address attention, relevance, confidence, and satisfaction.

14. To motivate learners, Biehler and Snowman suggest the use of

    A. textbooks.

    B. adventure.

    C. failure.

    D. society.

Rationale:

Biehler and Snowman ("Motivation," 1997) suggest the use of behavioral techniques, addressing what is required with the process and achievement, satisfying deficiency needs, emphasizing rewards and consequences, focusing on success, and having a sense of adventure.

15. Clinical simulation activities require the formation of a group to manage the client scenario. Which generational groups would function better in this type of learning situation?

    A. Veterans and Baby Boomer
    B. Baby Boomer and Millennial
    C. Veteran and Generation X
    D. Generation X and Millennial

Rationale:

The Veteran and Generation X cohorts want to work independently toward goals. Baby Boomers and Millennials value the benefits of teamwork to reach a goal/outcome.

16. To motivate Generation Xers, the faculty member should work to establish

    A. goals, then let them do it their own way.
    B. goals and paths for them to use.
    C. groups, then let them come up with their own goals.
    D. goals and stay with them to direct the process.

Rationale:

When endeavoring to motivate the Generation X group, it is wise to remember that they are self-starters and results-driven. Providing goals for them then getting out of their way to allow them to creatively and individually complete the goals is beneficial.

Discussion Questions

1. Design a model for evidence-based teaching in your setting.

Considerations:

- Future directions of nursing education
- Target audience characteristics
- Outcomes to achieve
- Evaluation of the model; how to test

2. What motivates the students in your program to learn?

Considerations:

- Identify generational characteristics.
- Identify strategies that students indicate motivate them.
- Explore strategies that are new/different from yours.
- Select a motivational theory that is relevant to your setting.

Teaching Scenario

1. You have been assigned to teach a nursing theory course. Nursing theories are considered by the students as abstract and having no relevance to nursing practice. How would you motivate the students to incorporate a nursing theory in their approach to nursing care? What evidence would you use to demonstrate the need for a relationship of theory to practice?

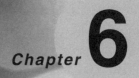

Chapter 6

Classroom Educational Experiences

Sharon Cannon

Chapter Objectives

At the conclusion of this chapter, the learner will be able to:

1. Trace the path of objectives from the organizational level to the unit level.
2. Identify effective teaching skills for the classroom.
3. Utilize management of classroom strategies.
4. Evaluate students in a classroom educational experience.

Key Terms

- ➤ Behavioral objective
- ➤ Bloom's taxonomy
- ➤ Case studies/problem-based learning
- ➤ Classroom assessment
- ➤ Classroom management
- ➤ Clickers
- ➤ Formative evaluation

- ➤ Muddiest points
- ➤ 1-minute papers
- ➤ PDAs
- ➤ Reflective journaling
- ➤ Role play
- ➤ Student evaluation
- ➤ Summative evaluation

Introduction

Historically, the traditional approach to teaching has been in the classroom. Though a significant shift occurred with the introduction of distance education, the classroom experience has and will continue to be a vital venue for teaching, regardless of the discipline/profession. Increased technology for the provision of content to motivate and engage the student in the learning process has impacted how faculty will involve students in the acquisition of knowledge. As a result, classroom experiences for the 21st century will move well beyond the "sage on the stage," lecture-only format (see Chapter 3). The classroom experience will involve much more than the faculty member giving a lecture and students dutifully taking notes.

Evidence-based teaching (EBT) has emerged from growing demands of students for involvement in the educational process. In light of economic changes, a diverse audience of learners exists. No longer are they only those who are straight from high school. Many are seeking a second career or deciding that perhaps now that children are in school, they can go back to college and pursue their dream of becoming a nurse. The diverse audience of learners, along with technological advances, requires innovation/creative approaches in the classroom. Consequently, faculty will need to examine closely the course/unit objectives, teaching strategies, and the management of the classroom experience. Together, these aspects culminate in evaluating the students' progress toward successfully acquiring the knowledge necessary. To accomplish such goals, faculty will need to acquire sophisticated skills useful in the classroom. Thus, the focus of this chapter is on providing multiple options for faculty to use in the classroom educational experience.

Behavioral Objectives

The essence of EBT is deeply embedded in **behavioral objectives**. The initial aspect of teaching requires a close look at behavioral objectives for the course being taught. It is important to realize that those objectives are part of a greater picture. To grasp the complexity of objectives, faculty must look further to the college/university, school, and program objectives (see **Figure 6-1**). Obviously, course objectives are just one of the building blocks for the whole educational experience. In addition, course objectives are broken down further into unit objectives. All of these objectives will eventually be evaluated throughout the educational process (see Chapter 9 regarding program evaluation). Ultimately the measure of success is reflected by students who complete all of the requirements by meeting objectives for graduation.

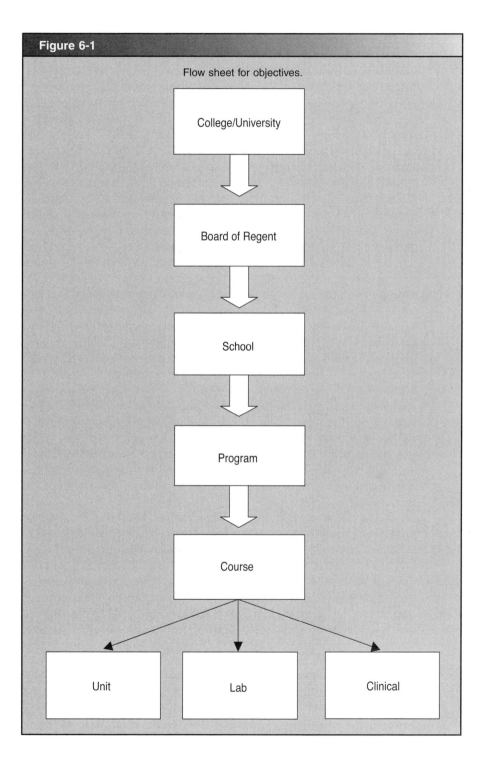

Figure 6-1

Flow sheet for objectives.

College/University

Board of Regent

School

Program

Course

Unit

Lab

Clinical

Perhaps, at this point, a distinction between a goal and an objective is necessary, as we hear a lot about goals related to schools and programs. Often a goal is thought to be an objective, and vice-versa. Some controversy exists, as others believe that goals and objectives are separate. A goal may be considered to be a broad statement of what is to be achieved. An objective is more specific and determines what is to be accomplished and by whom (Wingate, 2008). An example of a goal that is separated from an objective is: "The goal is to provide students with knowledge regarding genomics." A related objective would be "To provide genomics information in medical/surgical nursing in the Foundation of Nursing course offered in the first semester of the junior year and the Professional Nursing course taught in the last semester of the senior year." For this chapter, goals are considered as broad and objectives as specific.

As mentioned earlier, course objectives are often broken down to unit objectives to manage the presentation of content and from simple to complex levels of content. Regardless of whether the objectives are based on unit or course content, all objectives must be measureable. Remember objectives specify what and when content is to be learned. For instance, an objective that states, "The learner will understand fluid and electrolyte balance" is not measurable. The verb "understand" is broad, not specific, and has no criteria for measuring achievement. Instead, the faculty must spell out what behavior the student must display for comprehension about fluid and electrolyte balance. An example might be "The student will be able to differentiate the results of too much fluid and not enough potassium." This example is more specific and states the mechanism to indicate how the objective will be met. An important point to remember is that course and unit objectives are interrelated and drive the design of the educational experience.

To measure an objective, as stated before, the faculty must determine what behavior the student is to display. Thus, behavioral objectives are required. The seminal work on behavioral objectives began in 1956 when Dr. Benjamin Bloom published his taxonomy of educational objectives in cooperation with a group of educational psychologists including his mentor Ralph W. Tyler. **Bloom's Taxonomy** is considered the "gold standard" and hallmark of behavioral objectives and is divided into six levels of learning: recall, grasp, apply, analyze, synthesize, and judge. In addition, there are three domains where learning takes place: affective (feeling), cognitive (thinking), and psychomotor (acting). Bloom also thought the environment was important as well as the arrangement of how learning was to be promoted. It must be noted at this point that a controversy exists between the use of outcomes and competencies (Caputi, 2010). A more current emphasis in nursing education suggests that behavioral objectives are prescriptive and are unable to elicit more complex outcomes for higher levels of learning. This chapter offers faculty the opportunity to clarify their own opinions. Generally, faculty members are perceived to have control over the curriculum. Thus, it is extremely important for faculty to decide whether to use behavioral objectives, outcomes/competencies, or a modified approach to the design of the program and courses. Regardless of the faculty members' choices, it is important to consider that behavioral objectives are still very highly regarded and are used in most educational venues.

Bloom's taxonomy is widely utilized by nurse educators today in the development, implementation, and evaluation of objectives in the classroom environment. Entire textbooks have been written about the use of Bloom's Taxonomy, the details of which are beyond the scope of this chapter. However, all faculty members are highly recommended to study his work so that the behavioral objectives they use are measureable, involve the levels of learning, and are in the appropriate domain. Without this understanding, faculty will be unable to effectively teach and evaluate student outcomes, regardless of the learning environment, as behavioral objectives exist for more than the classroom (i.e., lab/simulation and clinical settings).

Teaching Strategies

Once the behavioral objectives have been determined for the course, unit, and environment, faculty must begin to address the content to be taught. A word of caution must be given here. Faculty cannot teach everything there is to know, nor is it appropriate to do so. Time is also a factor. Each course has only so much time allowed for the content to be presented. The type of program (undergraduate or graduate), level of the student learner (junior, senior, or generational category), physical environment (classroom, online, lab, or clinical) must also be considered. Trying to teach everything can be frustrating for both faculty and students, and, needless to say, impossible to accomplish in the given time constraints, regardless of the setting. It is essential that faculty focus on what the student needs to know rather than what would be nice (great) for the student to know in the time allowed. Rushing through content will not always allow students to master content and ultimately will overwhelm the student. Bloom recognized that speed is not the issue, especially to achieve measurable educational objectives and goals. Time to reflect, analyze, and synthesize are important.

Now that objectives have been made measurable and content has been specified, delivery methods must be determined. Whether to lecture or not to lecture may be the question. Traditionally, the lecture format has been the standard. With the advent of adult learning and motivational theories of learning along with advanced technology (see Chapter 3), teaching strategies have become diverse. In fact, some faculty members perceive the available strategies to be an open field and use multiple approaches for teaching in the classroom.

Since the lecture strategy is probably the most widely used, let's look at what options an effective lecture mode should incorporate. Generally, experienced faculty start by dividing content in units and then outlining each unit to be taught. The next step is finding references for the specific content as well as capitalizing on the expertise of the faculty who will be lecturing. Following that step is the need to determine what resources may be used. For example, faculty may choose to use PowerPoint, videos, or CD recordings, or a combination of these. Questions and discussion time will also need to be added. Other items to be considered for the classroom include the use of PDAs, clickers, case studies or problem-based learning, 1-minute papers and muddiest points, and role play, each of which is discussed later in this chapter.

Recognizing that different generations of students are in the class, a variety of approaches may be necessary to facilitate each student's grasp of the content being presented. Using a variety of approaches in the classroom plays an important part in motivating students, stimulating thoughts/ideas, and making content (which can be very dry and technical at times) more interesting and applicable to the students' experiences. All of these points should be addressed before you prepare to teach in a classroom. Remember that there is absolutely nothing more boring than for a faculty member to stand in front of a class and read his or her lecture notes. Motivating, engaging, and energizing students in the learning process is essential to achieve the objectives for the unit and the course. As Bloom indicated, the learning process is more than recalling information. Nursing faculty who are engaged in eliciting critical thinking must provide opportunities for higher levels of learning in dynamic teaching approaches. This will require faculty to select the best teaching strategy and to be adept in utilizing a variety of technology approaches.

Managing the Classroom Environment

In **classroom management**, two primary considerations must be addressed. The first is to manage the size of the class. Obviously, strategies used for teaching 30 students will differ greatly from those used when teaching 100-plus students. The greater the size of the class, the less likely it is to have all students actively participate in class activities. The second consideration is the number of faculty to teach the course.

Sometimes with very large classes only one faculty member may present content, or a teaching assistant (TA) might help. Other classes may involve guest speakers or have several faculty members assigned to assist with content. The faculty members assigned primary responsibility must realize the advantages and disadvantages of small/large class size to manage the class.

Once the objectives have been established and the teaching modalities selected, faculty must determine how to manage the classroom. Coyle-Rogers (2008) suggests that the classroom has a physical and psychological environment that impacts the relationship between the faculty and students. Creating a positive, supportive, respectful, and diverse environment leads to maximum communication and influences learning outcomes. Coyle-Rogers (2008) notes seating arrangements, the setting of expectations, faculty and student preparation, and teacher strategies such as eye contact, tone of voice, personality, and even physical appearance/demeanor as important considerations. Other aspects include room size, temperature, audio equipment, props, handouts, and overall organization of content and activities. Faculty must promote participation from at least a majority of students, with all being engaged as the ultimate goal. Creating a positive environment is powerful and requires faculty to coordinate complex strategies to facilitate learning.

Wingate (2008) looks more closely at classroom management. She starts by examining pre-lecture nerves, which many novice and experienced faculty experience. Not everyone desires being in the spotlight, and some may feel anxious before standing in front of a room full of students who may be younger, older, or the same age as the faculty. Loving the subject you teach and being prepared may alleviate some anxiety. Worthy to note is that though you may present as an authority on the subject, you do not need to have all the answers. It is okay and even preferable to say "I don't know" as long as you state "I'll find out" or prompt the class to find resources providing the answer. Obviously, you cannot reply "I don't know" to every question, but you can also be a role model to students when you explore options for learning for yourself and others. Students are less apt to "bluff" their way through a situation where "knowing" impacts the patient's outcome. Master teachers often express they would rather have a student/nurse say "I don't know but I'll find out" than cause harm to a patient.

Another aspect of classroom management is getting students to pay attention. This can be a daunting task. With cell phones, i-phones, and students talking to one another, the noise levels and lack of attentiveness becomes almost chaotic. Most schools have policies regarding cell phones and i-phones, so faculty should become familiar with and enforce such policies in the classroom. As for students conversing with one another, faculty may have to confront the problem individuals, which becomes extremely uncomfortable for everyone. Some ideas to counteract the discomfort are to randomly assign seats so that student groups are not together. You can also stop talking and wait, suggest they write notes to each other, ask for courtesy to others, stand next to those talking, or simply ask the individuals to share their comments with the class.

If you notice the students aren't being attentive, you might change the tone of your voice, make sure the audio equipment is working, walk around, or change the pace of the lecture. Another suggestion is to be aware of how long students have been sitting. If you are doing a 3-hour lecture, you need to allow for a 10- to 15-minute break at least one or two times. Sometimes just having students stand and stretch even though it is not break time allows them to be able to focus. Remember that classes were originally designed for 50 minutes because that is about the maximum for an effective attention span.

Another aspect to address is the name/title you wish to be called and whether students prefer to be addressed by their first or last name. This allows for respect to be a two-way street and shows concern so that students know you care about them. Some doctorally prepared faculty wish for students to address them as Dr. (last name). Others don't want to be that formal. By the same token, older students may prefer that you use their last name. Some students may use their middle name rather then their first name. The idea is to promote an environment that is courteous, respectful, and yet comfortable for both faculty and students.

Getting students to answer correctly, especially with difficult concepts, can be a challenge. It is extremely important not to embarrass a student. So if the student answers incorrectly, you might rephrase the question or give an example of what kind of response you expect. Perhaps you can allow the students to use a **PDA** or the Internet to find the answer if PDAs or computers are accessible, and then allow the students to report back to the class with the correct information. Again, be sure that you are supportive and have laid the groundwork so that it is okay to be wrong as long as the correct information is sought and obtained.

Games and **role playing** create a more participative learning experience that can be incorporated into lectures. Along with **case studies** and **problem-based learning** are ways to promote critical thinking and collaborative learning. A game of Jeopardy, a crossword puzzle, and Trivial Pursuit are ideas that have elicited class participation. Faculty who wish to incorporate games or establish roles for students to play should search the literature for ideas. Some faculty members even create their own games and use them very effectively.

As can be seen, lecturing and managing the classroom require much thought and preparation. The traditional lecture has gone far beyond faculty presenting content and students taking notes. The "sage on the stage" model is still present, but alternatives are available to engage students in the learning process. To make sure that you have been successful, the next step is to do a classroom assessment. It is not enough to be creative, innovative, or even entertaining if classroom instruction and student learning do not take place.

Classroom Assessment

Rowles (2009) recommended to use the definition of Angels (1994, p. 5) to define **classroom assessment** as the following: "consists of small scale assessments conducted continuously in the college classroom by discipline-based teachers to determine what students are learning in that class" (p. 262). A classroom assessment promotes learning as the class progresses and the faculty member uses techniques to facilitate learning. Thus, you will encounter CATs (Classroom Assessment Techniques) in the literature. CATs are formative in nature. **Formative evaluations** are the ongoing, periodical, and routine assessments done throughout a course (for more information on formative evaluation, see Chapter 9). CATs provide immediate feedback that faculty can use to determine if they are on track and students are comprehending content. This information can then allow opportunities for faculty to reflect on and change their teaching where appropriate. In addition, students can be more interactive and discover their own individual gaps in knowledge, affirm the knowledge they have gained, or clarify areas that are unclear. Examples of CATs are the 1-minute paper, muddiest points, and clickers. The **1-minute paper** requires student to write a maximum of a half a page in 5 minutes to answer one question: What was the most important thing you learned today? The **Muddiest point** may also be done as a 1-minute paper where the student has to write the most confusing point on a half a page in 5 minutes. **Clickers** are considered to be a type of audience response system (ARS). Faculty members poll student responses to a specific question. Students respond using a remote control device. The program tabulates the responses, and the faculty member then provides feedback to students. Using CATs allows faculty to improve teaching and learning activities while the course is in progress. This allows for adjustments during the course rather than after the course has been completed and provides for more positive outcomes for both faculty and students.

Student Evaluation

The ultimate determination of the successful classroom delivery modality is through **evaluation of the students**. Multiple approaches are available to assess whether students learn content provided throughout the classroom experience. The first thoughts that come to mind are those related to tests/examinations. A test provides a means for students to correct misinformation and identify specific gaps in knowledge. Tests also provide faculty with the tools to measure student progress, identify unclear areas of content, and evaluate desired outcomes for learning. Tests are closely connected to course objectives, which require faculty to be precise about content, time frame, and teaching/learning strategies for course content mastery. Consequently, tests must align with course objectives, be reliable (consistently produce the same results), and valid (actually/accurately measure the content). Many schools of nursing and even the National Council of State Boards establish a blueprint to provide a plan for selecting items for a test. Often the test blueprint is provided to students to assist them in studying and preparing for the exam.

There are a wide variety of options for formatting a test—multiple choice, true/false, matching, fill in the blank, open ended, and essays. Experienced faculty members often use a variety of these formats to gain a more comprehensive view of students' progress. Test and measurement courses are highly recommended, especially for novice faculty, to obtain greater proficiency and confidence regarding the usage of various test formats and the level and/or domain of learning, such as comprehension, recall, or skill acquisition. Each testing format has a place in the evaluation of student progress.

Regardless of the test format, tests may be formative or summative. Tests used throughout the course are considered formative, usually concentrating on partial content such as a unit. Final comprehensive exams are considered **summative evaluations**, because they measure content presented over the entire course. Regardless of whether courses tests are formative or summative, tests enable students to become adept at taking tests, which also assists with taking standardized tests used for progression through the program, graduation, and ultimately the NCLEX exam to practice nursing.

With the advancement of technology and trends in nursing education, other options for evaluating students are available. Sheldon (2008) provides a menu of methods available for measuring student learning:

- Portfolios
- Group projects
- Role play
- Case studies
- Concept maps
- Concept papers
- **Reflective journaling**
- Research critiques
- Socratic questions
- Videotaping (p. 287)

Selection of the method of evaluation depends on multiple criteria: size of the class, the number of faculty teaching, setting (classroom, lab, or clinical), types of students (older/younger generation), resources (technology), and the nature of the course content, to name a few. Faculty must be knowledgeable about evaluation methods to select the most appropriate type of assessment.

The prior discussion has examined formative evaluation of students throughout a course. The final step of student evaluation involves summative evaluation. Summative evaluation is "done at the end of the semester or course to provide the final judgment as to whether or not the student has achieved the educational goals" (Oermann, Saewert, Charasika, & Yarbrough, 2009, p. 353). Grades accumulated in the formative evaluation must now culminate in a final grade. Some courses, especially clinical or lab courses, are a pass/fail. Most courses taught in the classroom assign grades based on a scale of A, B, C, D, or F. Depending on the faculty selection, the final grade earned by the student may be a compilation of the formative grades, a comprehensive exam, paper, and/or case study. Faculty must remember to be fair, consistent, and clear about the evaluation resulting in any grade assigned. If there are several faculty members teaching the course and responsible for a group of students within the course, interrater reliability must be established to maintain consistency, eliminate bias, and assure fairness for all students in the class. Students and faculty alike are often anxious about grading outcomes. Assuring consistency and fairness across the board can alleviate at least some of the stress associated with grades. Faculty and students want positive results from the evaluation process to eliminate biases.

Having mechanisms in place to ensure impartial grading and guidance throughout the course assists the student in achieving the course requirements. Unfortunately, reality is that not all students will be able to accomplish what is required. It would be wonderful if all students were to pass, but that is not always possible. Faculty will need to thoroughly review student evaluations of the course, test results, interrater reliability, peer reviews by other faculty who might teach the course, and appropriateness of objectives, teaching strategies, and resources used.

Summary Thoughts

The classroom educational experience is a dynamic, complex venue. An orchestra conductor has multiple musicians to manage just one single harmonious note as part of a total musical score. Faculty in the classroom environment must "orchestrate" the multiple aspects of teaching a course. Developing objectives, designing content presentation strategies, and evaluating student/course outcomes are indeed difficult. Advancements in technology and emerging trends in nursing education require nurse educators to adapt to changes that will be required in the new healthcare reform legislation. Traditional approaches to classroom teaching are being challenged to meet the demands of students, programs, employers of nurses, and the public. In fact, Benner, Sutphen, Leonard, and Day (2010) have called for a "radical transformation" in the classroom connected with the clinical setting through integrative teaching of knowledge, skills, and ethics.

The classroom experience may be the traditional lecture format. However, in today's nursing education milieu, lecture is not, and should not be, the only approach for acquisition of knowledge and skills. Many options are available to enhance student participation and performance in the classroom.

Linking course objectives to educational strategies and evaluation of students and the course are essential for managing the course. Ultimately, the classroom educational experience is an adaptable forum and an exciting environment for teaching and learning. Evaluations provide the evidence for effectiveness of teaching/learning in the classroom experience. Through evaluations, faculty who teach in that environment gain confidence that the acquisition of knowledge has occurred with positive outcomes for a student.

The classroom educational experience is a viable format for EBT. Faculty who use evidence for teaching/learning to guide delivery of content in the classroom can achieve successful outcomes for students and programs by employing diverse teaching strategies and using formative and summative evaluations. Feedback from multiple sources from students and peers enable faculty to effectively manage and evaluate the classroom experience.

Summary Points

1. Classroom experiences for the 21st century will move beyond the "sage on the stage," lecture-only format.
2. Evidence-based teaching has emerged from growing demands of students for involvement in the educational process.
3. Evidence-based teaching is deeply embedded in behavioral objectives.
4. An objective is specific and determines what is to be accomplished and by whom (Wingate, 2008).
5. A goal is a broad statement of what is to be achieved.
6. Recent literature reveals that controversy exists between the use of behavioral objectives versus outcomes and competencies (Caputi, 2010).
7. Institutions (universities/colleges), schools of nursing, nursing programs, and courses all have objectives that flow and are related to each other.
8. Courses objectives can be broken down to unit objectives as well as lab and clinical objectives, where appropriate.
9. Objectives measure the behavior the student is to display.
10. Dr. Benjamin Bloom published his taxonomy of educational objectives in 1956.
11. Bloom's taxonomy is used widely by nurse educators.
12. Multiple aspects impact the presentation of content to be taught.
13. A wide range of teaching/learning methods is available, such as PDAs, clickers, case studies/problem-based learning, muddiest points, and role playing.
14. Managing the classroom experience involves class size, physical/psychological aspects, faculty preparation, student participation, attendance, respect for faculty and students, and games/role playing.
15. Classroom assessment techniques (CATs) are considered formative evaluations implemented throughout the course.
16. Examples of CATs are one-minute papers, muddiest points, clickers, and examinations.
17. Student evaluations are both formative and summative.
18. Testing comes in several forms (i.e., multiple choice, true/false, matching, fill in the blanks, open ended, and essay).
19. With the advancement of technology and trends in nursing education, other options for evaluating students are available.
20. The final steps of evaluation of students include the individual performance of each student as well as student evaluations of the course.
21. The classroom educational experience is a dynamic, complex venue.
22. Benner, Sutphen, Leonard, and Day (2010) have called for a "radical transformation" of nursing education.
23. The classroom educational experience is an adaptable forum and an exciting environment for teaching and learning.
24. Evidence-based teaching can be accomplished in the classroom environment.

Tips for Nurse Educators to Use

1. Develop behavioral objectives that can be measured.
2. Use Bloom's Taxonomy to determine the level, type, and domain for learning to be achieved.
3. Focus on specific content to be covered in the time allotted.
4. Explore all options for delivery of content so that different generations of students will participate.
5. Consider class size, number of faculty teaching, and resources available.
6. Utilize effective classroom management techniques.
7. Analyze CATs for formative evaluation to identify gaps in knowledge, affirm knowledge gained, and clarify confusing/contradicting content.
8. Synthesize formative and summative student/course evaluations for trends and use the data (evidence) to improve the course taught in a classroom educational experience.

References

Benner, P., Sutphen, M., Leonard, V., & Day, L. (2010). *Educating nurses: A call for radical transformation.* San Francisco, CA: Jossey-Bass.

Caputi, L. (2010). Curriculum design and development. In L. Caputi (Ed.), *Teaching nursing: The art and science* (pp. 367–394). Glen Ellyn, IL: College of DuPage Press.

Coyle-Rogers, P. G. (2008). The power of the classroom climate. In B. K. Penn (Ed.), *Mastering the teaching role: A guide for nurse educators* (pp. 119–131). Philadelphia, PA: F.A. Davis.

Eisner, E. W. (2000). Benjamin Bloom. *Prospects: The quarterly review of comparative education,* XX(3). Paris, UNESCO: International Bureau of Education.

Oermann, M. H., Saewert, K. J., Charasika, M., & Yarbrough, S. S. (2009). Assessment and grading practices in schools of nursing: National survey findings part II. *Nursing Education Perspectives, 30*(6), 352–357.

Rowles, C. J. (2009). Improving teaching and learning: Classroom assessment techniques. In D. M. Billings & J. A. Halstead (Eds.), *Teaching in nursing: A guide for faculty* (3rd ed., pp. 262–267). St. Louis, MO: Saunders Elsevier.

Sheldon, D. P. (2008). Beyond testing: Other ways to evaluation learning. In B. K. Penn (Ed.), *Mastering the teaching role: a guide for nurse educators* (pp. 287–298), Philadelphia, PA: F.A. Davis.

Wingate, A. (2008). Managing the modern classroom. In B. K. Penn (Ed.), *Mastering the teaching role: A guide for nurse educators* (pp. 133–152). Philadelphia, PA: F.A. Davis.

Web Links

View Bloom's taxonomy at http://hs.riverdale.K12.or.us/~dthompso/exhibition/ blooms.htm.

Multiple Choice Questions

1. For the 21st century, lecture will:
   A. Be the only delivery format.
   B. Be delivered only by the "sage on the stage."
   C. involve more than faculty lecturing with students taking notes.
   D. be obsolete.

Rationale:

In the 21st century, classroom experiences will move beyond the "sage on the stage" and involve more than faculty lecturing with students dutifully taking notes, instead using technological advancements and more interactive activities to facilitate student learning.

2. Evidence-based teaching has emerged due to
   A. student demands, economic changes, and a diverse audience of learners.
   B. the abundance of nursing education research to provide data for effective teaching.
   C. the fact that classroom educational experiences have not been effective.
   D. parental concerns that their child is not receiving the best education.

Rationale:

Evidence-based teaching has emerged from growing demands of students for involvement in the educational process. In light of economic changes, a diverse audience of learners exists.

3. Objectives measure what _____ the student is to display:
   A. personality
   B. behavior
   C. attitude
   D. understanding

Rationale:

To measure an objective, the faculty must determine what behavior is to be displayed by students.

4. A goal is considered to be:
   A. narrow.
   B. specific.
   C. timely.
   D. broad.

Rationale:

A goal may be considered as a broad statement of what is to be achieved.

5. When determining content to be taught, faculty must consider:
   A. personal preferences, physical environment, and time.
   B. **type of program, time allotted, and levels of the students**.
   C. speed of delivery, personality of students, and size of the podium.
   D. personal preferences, size of the podium, and levels of the students.

Rationale:

Time is a factor. The type of program (undergraduate or graduate), level of the learner (junior, senior, or generational category), and physical environment (classroom, online, lab, or clinical) must also be considered.

6. Instructional methodology for the educational classroom experience may include:
   A. **lecture, PowerPoint slides, videos, and/or CD recordings**.
   B. lecture, PowerPoint slides, and/or chats.
   C. chats, discussion board messages, and/or animated cartoons.
   D. note taking, chats, and/or guest lecturers.

Rationale:

Faculty may choose to use lecture, PowerPoint slides, videos, and/or CD recordings, or a combination of these.

7. To be effective lecturers, faculty members should:
   A. read from their notes.
   B. ignore room size.
   C. speak in a quiet/low tone of voice.
   D. **use a variety of approaches**.

Rationale:

Using a variety of approaches may be necessary to facilitate a student's grasp of the content being presented.

8. Attendance requirements for a class should involve:
   A. the student's preference.
   B. the faculty's preference.
   C. **the school's/program's policy**.
   D. none of the above.

Rationale:

Faculty need to be sure of the school's/program's policy regarding attendance.

9. Critical thinking or problem solving can be:
   A. **accomplished through games and role playing**.
   B. accomplished through recall and memorization.

C. dull and boring.

D. impossible to achieve in the classroom.

Rationale:

Games and role playing create a more participative learning experience that can be incorporated into lecture. They are ways to promote critical thinking or solutions to problems posed as case studies.

10. Classroom Assessment Techniques (CATs) are:

A. summative.

B. final.

C. useless.

D. formative.

Rationale:

CATs are formative in nature.

11. Student evaluations may consist of:

A. tests.

B. portfolios.

C. journals.

D. all of the above.

Rationale:

Multiple approaches are available to assess whether students learn content provided through the classroom experience.

12. Final course grades are based on:

A. comprehensive exams only.

B. compilation of formative grades.

C. administrator decisions.

D. student requests.

Rationale:

Depending on the faculty selection, the final grade earned by the student may be a compilation of formative grades, a comprehensive exam, papers, and/or case study discussions.

13. Bias in grading when several faculty are involved can be eliminated by:

A. interrater reliability.

B. faculty popularity.

C. student popularity.

D. none of the above.

Rationale:

If there are several faculty teaching the course and responsible for a group of students within the course, interrater reliability must be established to maintain consistency, eliminate bias, and assure fairness for all students in the class.

14. The classroom educational experience is:

A. rigid and set in stone.
B. loose and free in requirements.
C. adaptable and exciting.
D. dull and boring.

Rationale:

Ultimately, the classroom educational experience is an adaptable forum and an exciting environment for teaching and learning.

Discussion Questions

1. You have been assigned to teach a nursing research course in a newly established undergraduate nursing program. How will you develop the course objectives?

Considerations:

- What are the program objectives?
- How many objectives does the course need to have?
- Will you use Bloom's Taxonomy or an outcome and competency approach?
- What behaviors/indicators will students need to display?
- How will you measure each objective?

2. You have been assigned the lead instructor role for team teaching a Foundations in Nursing class composed of 130 students. How will you manage the course?

Considerations:

- How many other faculty will teach?
- What is the expertise/clinical background of each faculty member?
- What responsibility does each faculty have (e.g., grading, simulation/lab, clinical, etc.)?
- Which teaching strategies will be chosen?
- What formative/summative evaluations will be used?

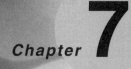

Online Educational Experiences

Carol Boswell

Chapter Objectives

At the conclusion of this chapter, the learner will be able to:

1. Compare different types of teaching strategies effective within an online educational experience.
2. Contrast aspects related to the delivery of online learning.
3. Discuss operational technology utilized in online teaching settings.
4. Examine strategies associated with evaluations resulting from online delivery of the educational process.

Key Terms

➤ Asynchronous activities

➤ Computer-based instruction

➤ Distance learners

➤ E-books

➤ Emoticons

➤ Engaged learning

➤ Face-to-face

➤ Netiquette rules

➤ Online courses

➤ Synchronous activities

➤ Technology

➤ Web-based instruction

Introduction

With the changing demographics related to health care, the need and expectation to engage in innovative methods of education become increasingly significant. According to the National Sample Survey of Registered Nurses (NSSRN) (U.S. Department of Health and Human Services, Health Resources and Services Administration [DHHS], 2010), the percentage of RNs employed full time increased from 58.4% (2004) to 63.2% (2008). This increasing percentage of RNs working full time may be attributed to the economy issues confronting the United States, but it must be noted that these data were collected prior to 2008. The economic recession happened in 2008, with the beginning effects of the downturn occurring for several years prior to this crash. Some of the speculation within the nursing community has centered on the idea that nurses who had anticipated retiring have remained in the workforce at this point due to family economic conditions. During this same time period (2004–2008), the number of nurses with an associate's degree (AD) rose from 42.9% to 45.4% (DHHS, 2010). Another concerning statistic identified by the NSSRN data shows that the share of nurses who are under the age of 40 currently is 29.5%, which is a slight increase from prior years (DHHS, 2010), but still remains low. The statistics suggest "among nurses 55 and older, 76,915 intend to leave the nursing profession within 3 years; another 54,539 intend to leave their current nursing job and are unsure if they will remain in nursing afterward" (DHHS, 2010, p. 10). With just these statistical considerations, the need to develop and implement creative ways to further education for the next generations of nurses takes on increasing importance.

Nurses who are prepared at the AD level are working more, thus they cannot (or will not) take off work to attend traditionally offered RN-BSN programs. According to the Tri-Council for Nursing (2010), "a more highly educated nursing profession is no longer a preferred future; it is a necessary future in order to meet the nursing needs of the nation and to deliver effective and safe care" (p. 1). With the push toward Magnet or Pathway to Excellence status by hospitals, the need for advancement of the AD registered nurses to the BSN level of education is strongly desired. Even with this cry to increase the educational preparation levels of registered nurses, agencies are focused on strictly controlling costs. Academic institutions are also confronted with the demand to reduce costs. As a result, dynamic online educational opportunities are viewed as an innovative, cost-effective approach (see Table 7-1). Connors (2008) noted, "today's students approach academics with a set purpose: a desire for efficiency in learning, a perception of what they need to learn and, most important, a planned set of outcomes" (p. 164). Generation X and Millennial

Table 7-1
Strengths Associated with Online Learning by Students
• The process is interactive and reinforces class content. • Online learning allows students the opportunity to apply theory to practice. • Nursing curriculum can be developed to use a combination of required and optional assignments. • Online learning accommodates the different learning styles when set up appropriately.
Source: Adapted from Noel-Levitz. (2006). *National online learner priorities report.* Braintree, MA: Author; and Leski, J. (2009). Nursing students and faculty perceptions of computer-based instruction at a 2-year college. *Journal of Nursing Education, 48*(2), 91–95.

cohorts want a learning environment that is accessible, flexible, learner-centered, and meshes with their lifestyle and commitments. Designers of programs of study need to carefully consider the manner in which the courses are presented and managed. Faculty members must take care to ensure that the students can stay true to their need to be individuals and open to fun.

As the movement toward online educational tactics is considered, care must be given to the evidence available concerning the optimal techniques necessary to be effective and successful. Draves (2000) makes a good point that "learning is not purely a cognitive process, but that it also involves the emotions and even the spirit" (p. 10). This chapter will endeavor to present key aspects related to online teaching. These aspects can then be carefully and thoroughly considered as decisions related to online delivery methods are made.

Types of Teaching Strategies

Several terms related to online education need to be defined to establish a foundation on which to build a body of understanding about the technique. According to Connors (2008), "distance education is organized education that occurs when the teacher and the learner are not in the same physical space at the same time" (p. 163). Thus, the term *distance education* is basically self-explanatory. Bastable (2003) lists examples of distance learning as online courses (discussed later in the chapter), correspondence courses, independent study, and videoconferencing. Whenever the teacher and the students (learners) are not in the same location, this term is applicable. Draves (2000) states that the characteristics of online learning include: "content is delivered differently, learners have to initiate learning and actively go get it, a learner has to figure out what you want to learn, it takes self-direction, learning online is work, and it is outcome and results oriented" (p. 30). Each and every aspect within the delivery of the material is changed, thus providing challenges for the faculty member to ensure that each student receives the needed direction to be successful.

Palloff and Pratt (1999) bring up a very important aspect in regard to distance education when they champion the idea that consideration must be directed toward the development of community for the participants to facilitate the learning environment. The learners who elect to engage in the educational process from a distance, or **distance learners**, are frequently compelled to do it as a result of time, geographic, financial, or other constraints that restrict their ability to attend traditional classes. The distance learning environment is viewed as convenient, accessible, and flexible. Bangert and Easterby (2008) state that "the flexibility and convenience offered by Internet-based nursing programs has been an important strategy for addressing the critical shortage of baccalaureate and advanced registered nurse practitioners" (p. 54S). Distance education is viewed as a resourceful and professional alternate for acquiring an advanced degree during these economic times, as it eliminates travel to a traditional classroom setting. Distance education is also coming to the forefront due to the surge of members from the Nexter Generation, who are technologically advanced.

A second key term central to distance learning is **technology**. Within the realm of online delivery methodology, any venue or device that allows students and faculty members to engage in the learning process from unique locations can be used. While the computer and Internet tend to be the most frequently utilized aspects, other devices are being incorporated as technology grows and develops. The Internet tends to be the only access point, but multiple devices are now being used in place of the computer. iPods, teleconferencing, cell phones, and readers are just a few of the devices that are becoming increasingly important in the world of online education.

Another term used within online learning is **engaged learning**. According to Conrad and Donaldson (2004), "engaged learning is focused on the learner, whose role is integral to the generation of new knowledge" (p. 5). Engaged learning requires the learner to become directly involved in the entire learning process. The learner is an active participant in the process instead of the passive participant, which can occur within the traditional education setting. Each member within an online learning environment must connect to the material presented.

Other terms used within online education include face-to-face, synchronous activities, asynchronous activities, web-based instruction, online courses, computer-based instruction (CBI), e-books, and netiquette rules, each of which is discussed next. As each of these concepts is pulled together, an inclusive view of aspects within online educational experiences can be developed.

Face-to-face is the term applied to traditional classroom experiences. This term is used to depict the opportunity to be one-on-one with the student. With face-to-face educational experiences, faculty members are able to incorporate all of the senses in the process of educating the individual. Both nonverbal and verbal communication activities are utilized within the process. Nonverbal communication takes on a different flavor with online teaching. With the use of **emoticons**, or symbols that convey feelings, some of the aspects of nonverbal communication can come into play. As use of online education and texting have increased with the technologically advanced generations, multiple signs and abbreviations have been developed that take the place of nonverbal communication. Examples of such emoticons are: ☺, :-<, LOL (laugh out loud), BFF (best friends forever), and so forth. Within each course, students need to be careful, as some faculty members do not allow the use of these nonverbal communication graphics. New abbreviations and graphics constantly are added to the online communication, which allows individuals to see the nonverbal feelings of the other participants. But within the online community, this process is limited. Participants must willfully engage in the documenting of their nonverbal communication, whereas in the classroom, the members of the classroom can look around and view the nonverbal communication of their classmates. In the face-to-face environment, the participants do not have to wait for colleagues to engage in documenting their nonverbal feelings—such communication is readily apparent. Within the online community, participants can remain neutral if desired. If a peer does not convey such information deliberately, the primary indication that a problem is developing may only be the decrease in communication connectiveness by that individual.

Web-based instruction is any activity/course which is provided via the Internet, and thus **online course** is a synonymous term. Lowenstein and Bradshaw (2004) denote the different ways to provide web-based instruction as:

- Totally web-based asynchronous (no face-to-face or real-time interaction);
- Totally web-based synchronous (no face-to-face interaction but class meets online in real time);
- Partially web-based with some face-to-face class meetings (plus asynchronous or synchronous class interactions); or
- A traditional class with supplemental web-based components (emails, forums, chat rooms, class content). (p. 210)

Each of these different methods allows for the individualization of the course. A faculty member can elect to use different levels of web-based instruction within a course presentation. The determination of the manner in which the course is delivered should be based on the needs of the student, content to be delivered, mission of the course/

program, and expectations of the learning community. Lowenstein and Bradshaw (2004) postulate that "participation in any form of distance learning requires students to be self-directed and able to function in an environment with limited faculty feedback and lacking face-to-face interaction" (p. 213). Students who engage in distance learning opportunities must understand that the responsibility for learning does fall upon them because they don't have the classroom to use for passive learning. Web-based instruction requires active learning and engagement in the learning process by the individual student.

Synchronous activities are those planned activities where all of the members are expected to be online and/or connected at the same time. These activities include chat room discussions, webinar activities, teleconferencing experiences, and so forth. The assigned individuals are compelled to be online with the other designated members at the same time. During these activities, the educational proceedings are completed during the designated time period, with everyone engaged in the learning process during that assigned time period.

The opposite of such activities is **asynchronous activities**. Asynchronous activities are viewed as those encounters that are conducted independently of other learners. Within this process, the learner can address the activity within the course at a time convenient for the individual. Asynchronous activities are done usually within a time period but not needing the direct attention of others. Discussion (bulletin) boards are an example of this type of activity. Assignments are made for students to post a specific number of messages within a designated time period. The student can determine when during that designated period to complete the assignment. The assignments/ postings are not done at the same time for all of the participants. The requirement is for the activity to be successfully done during the assigned time period. Any activity within the course that does not require the cohort to be together in the course shell at the same time but can be done at the convenience of the participant is asynchronous in nature.

Computer-based instruction (CBI) is a term used to denote any activities conducted on a computer for the acquisition of knowledge. From evidence, Leski (2009) noted that CBI:

- Pertains to specific content areas;
- Presents realistic demands on participants;
- Transpires in a setting with nominal disruption;
- Is time bound;
- Enhances learning under specified key circumstances;
- Hinders learning under specific central situations;
- Varies in application depending on a diversity of concerns; and
- Facilitates nursing education in specific spheres.

Computer-based instruction is functional for some areas but inappropriate for other areas. Topics that require hands-on management pose difficulty when considered for presentation via a computer-based delivery methodology.

E-books are gaining in attention and utilization within the learning process. E-books are presented on a computer instead of requiring the purchasing of hard copies or printed textbooks. Several advantages can be considered as a result of using e-books. According to Williams and Dittmer (2009), "the bundled e-book package was handier to use than several books, and students felt that the e-book information gave them extra confidence" (p. 224). The computer-based delivery of books allows for a quick turnaround when updates are needed. The cost of the books is reduced because time and resources are not used. The environment is also saved because the books do not require printing, thus saving of our trees. In addition, students can access the books for resources when in a clinical setting. "It is important for educators and librarians to take note of the different information retrieval styles of new generations of learners" (Williams & Dittmer, 2009, p. 224). Since the books are accessed via the computer or iPod devices, a question can be quickly researched to determine up-to-date information when making critical decisions.

A final term to consider in regard to online courses is the idea of **netiquette rules**. As the Internet has developed and expanded, individuals have pulled together concepts submitted as proper methods for engagement via online communication. These rules/recommendations cover the use of capital letters (to be avoided in most situations), proper use of the computer, management of emails, and so forth. Netiquette is viewed as the behaviors that reflect being civilized on the computer, similar to etiquette in a face-to-face setting.

General Aspects in Delivery of Online Education

Chickering and Gamson (1987) stated that effective management of the undergraduate educational experience required the encouraging of connection concerning students and faculty, cultivating teamwork among students, advancing vigorous learning, providing timely feedback, articulating quality expectations, and recognizing distinct techniques of learning. Within any educational setting, the need to present an effective and successful environment which encourages and showcases learning is of paramount importance. As education moves forward with online delivery, several aspects are essential to consider. Chickering and Gamson (1987) identified the areas of shared purposes, positive support by the administration, appropriate funding for the online delivery, policies and procedures that address the process of online delivery, and support for faculty members' development as they learn to conduct online education as keys for successful management of the online processes. Another area to carefully address within this area is the need for technology support on a 24-hour, 7-days-a-week basis for both the students and faculty members. Everyone within the educational setting needs to be on target for getting the different aspects of the process done successfully with quality outcomes.

As academic facilities consider providing online education, one initial aspect is the formation of the learning community. Since students are not sitting in the room with their colleagues and the faculty member, attention to methods for allowing the individuals within the course to connect as a learning community is of paramount importance. According to Palloff and Pratt (1999), "the keys to the creation of a learning community and successful facilitation online are simple— honesty, responsiveness, relevance, respect, openness, and empowerment" (p. 20). Taking the time to plan how to unite the different members in the course cohort is a critical foundation for the development of discussion and interactions. Since the individuals don't have the advantage of sitting in a room together, the development of a comfort level with the different individuals must take place through the use of communication skills (see Table 7-2). Bastable (2003) discusses the expectation that online courses need to facilitate learning activities and resources supporting teacher–learner and learner–learner interactions. Each aspect within the course must be painstakingly considered as to how it will lend itself to the formation of a learning community.

Dorin (2009) states, "online classes require a time commitment that's similar to that of classes in a traditional university—minus the commute!" (p. 35). Each aspect of the course reflects the openness of the presentation. Since accessing the course is flexible and convenient, the incorporation of assignments needs to flow from the beginning to the end. With online courses breaking out of the mold used for

Table 7-2
Top Challenges Associated with Online Learning by Students
• The quality of the instructional delivery for courses. • Staying attuned to the needs of the student cohort. • Timely and positive feedback to the students. • Not having enough time for deliberation and consideration by students of the content needed for the assignments. • Lack of time for grading by faculty. • Having issues with trust and freedom of expression when assigned reflective journaling.
Source: Adapted from Noel-Levitz. (2006). *National online learner priorities report.* Braintree, MA: Author; and Langley, M. E., & Brown, S. T. (2010). Perceptions of the use of reflective learning journals in online graduate nursing education. *Nursing Education Perspective, 31*(1), 12–17.

face-to-face classes, such courses need to justify the number of semester credit hours awarded with the work to be completed. Given that the courses depend on self-learning, assignments usually require readings, participation, and one other type of assignment per week. The assignments could involve papers, PowerPoint presentations, tests, or tutorials. The activities can entail actions accomplished individually or within teams.

Conrad and Donaldson (2004) suggest that "to determine whether a classroom-based activity is adaptable to the online environment, the activity must first be examined to see that it meets the learning outcomes of the online course" (p. 17). Learning objectives are the underpinning for the educational experience; thus, each and every activity to be incorporated into a course needs to be scrutinized to determine its functionality. Most face-to-face activities can be modified for use within the online delivery venue. Brainstorming is one type of activity that can be modified into an online assignment. When adapting this activity, the online "shout out" phrase would be the quick listing of key ideas within the subject line; everyone can quickly identify themes without having to open the documents. Other activities successfully used in face-to-face settings must be analyzed to see how they could be adapted for use in an online delivery venue.

Loyola (2010) looks at online education from the focus of outcome-based education. Outcome-based education "is a paradigm shift from passive traditional learning to an active, learner-centered, result-oriented approach to learning" (Loyola, 2010, p. 19). While any type of education can provide outcome-based education, online delivery is ripe for providing learning experiences that require the active participation of the learner. In regard to education being results-oriented, any educational experience must address the results to be obtained. To be effective, the teacher should determine the results expected from the engagement in the learning process. Loyola (2010) recommends that the faculty member must establish an educational milieu that is appealing, exciting, motivating, stimulating, and sustainable. The educator is responsible for the outcomes and conclusions resulting from the learning experience. Another aspect of teaching online relates to being able to effectively summarize. Loyola (2010) states "the learner must delete some information (trivial and redundant), substitute some information, and keep some information" (p. 23). This process of summarizing within an online course mandates that the participant scrutinize and dissect the content to a moderately multifaceted and meaningful degree. Superficial scrutiny of the material presented does not allow for the full acquisition of the content to be assimilated from the course. Within online delivery, this process of scrutinizing the information falls to the participants, rather than relying on the summary to be provided by the instructor during the class period. This process of driving the participant to dig deeper and analyze the different components within a topic encourages the participants to synthesize the material. It becomes a part of the student's knowledge basis. One final aspect is the need to focus attention during online education toward appropriate use of recognition and praise that indicates a higher level of learning. "Effective recognition needs to be positive and sincere in nature, immediately connected to performance, and specific about what is being praised" (Loyola, 2010, p. 23). Since a faculty member is not directly with the students, the need for recognition and immediacy is increased. Face-to-face delivery allows the faculty member to watch the verbal and nonverbal communication and engage accordingly. An online format does not allow this expediency related to encouragement and recognition. Faculty members need to contemplate when and how to provide recognition and encouragement that is timely and directed.

Draves (2000) suggests online education can outshine classroom learning because "a learner can: learn during her or his peak learning time, learn during her or his own speed, focus on specific content areas, test himself daily, and interact more with the teacher" (p. 11). Online delivery of educational experiences places a lot of the responsibility squarely on the learner. By making learners responsible for the acquisition of the material, the faculty member can focus on the delivery of the material. The delivery methods are very important, as they are the process by which the learner engages and acquires the information (see Table 7-3). Draves (2000) states a key aspect: "The heart and soul of an online course will be the interaction between the participants and teacher, as well as the interaction among the participants themselves" (p. 12). The faculty member must establish multiple venues for granting access to peers and faculty. Since the delivery is online and not face-to-face, every opportunity for engaging the participants (students and faculty) must be provided and encouraged. The opportunities to engage with peers and the faculty are the aspect that connects the individuals together in the learning process and aids in the networking for the members of the cohort involved in the online sessions.

One of the key aspects embedded in an online delivery system is the need to have effective communication. Hanna, Glowacki-Dudka, and Conceicao-Runlee (2000) describe "a learning community is a group of people who have come together to form a culture of learning in which everyone is involved in a collective effort of understanding" (p. 14). The development of this learning community requires that attention be given to the development and management of the communication between the members of the community. Online sessions move rapidly and require each member of the cohort to be self-disciplined and engaged. When members are not committed to the learning process, their delays can adversely affect the rest of the cohort. Discussion within the course requires that all members hold

Table 7-3

Suggestions When Planning and Conducting Online Courses

- Course content and delivery must be prepared in advanced.
- Students must be willing and encouraged to ask questions as needed.
- All aspects of the course should promote dialogue between the participants in the course—both students and faculty members.
- Participants within each course should be encouraged to examine their own learning process at regular intervals.
- Each online course should have at least three central components—subject matter, exchange, and appraisal.
- Using between 5 and 10 units/modules provides adequate division for a course.
- "A rough measurement for reading time is 20 pages an hour for nonfiction, 10 pages an hour for extremely technical information, and 40 pages an hour for fiction" (Draves, 2000, p. 79).
- Faculty members must learn to "chunk" materials because reading long narratives does not effectively encourage engagement and learning.
- Bullets and narratives within an online document should be kept short—approximately 6 to 8 lines of copy is a rule of thumb.
- "The one-minute assessment allows you to ask questions electronically and collect answers anonymously (if you have a program that allows learners to send responses anonymously)" (Hanna et al. 2000, p. 46).
- "A bulletin board, chat room, or threaded discussion can be developed for use by a specific class. Choice of communication method also depends on the need for group interaction, peer-to-peer interaction, or student-to-instructor interaction" (Lowenstein & Bradshaw, 2004, p. 199).
- "There is a skill to asking the 'right questions' to improve higher-level thinking. 'How' and 'why' questions usually require more analysis than 'who,' 'what,' 'when,' or 'where' questions" (Loyola, 2010, p. 27)
- The learners must participate in the class at least every other day to ensure connectedness.
- Instructional proficiency requires time management and boundary setting while constructing an online learning community.
- Fair use of materials within an online course involves an understanding of copyright law, which allows for regulated inclusion of copyrighted material without the owner's permission. A 10% rule advocates the use of 10% or less of a complete material as reasonable use.
- "Students who were assigned to facilitate commented that they learned more when they facilitated discussions than those for which they were not assigned that role" (Dell et al., 2010, para. 4).

Source: Adapted from Dell, C. A., Low, C., & Wilker, J. F. (2010). Comparing student achievement in online and face-to-face class formats. *Journal of Online Learning and Teaching 6*(1). Retrieved May 14, 2010 from http://jolt.merlot.org/vol6no1/dell_0310.htm; Draves, W. A. (2000). *Teaching online.* River Falls, WI: LERN books; Hanna, D. E., Glowacki-Dudka, M., & Conceicao-Runlee, S. (2000). *147 practical tips for teaching online groups: Essentials of web-based education.* Madison, WI: Atwood Publishing; Lowenstein, A. J. & Bradshaw, M. J. (2004). *Fuszard's innovative teaching strategies in nursing* (3rd ed.). Sudbury, MA: Jones and Bartlett Publishers; and Loyola, S. (2010). Evidence-based teaching guidelines: Transforming knowledge into practice for better outcomes in healthcare. *Critical Care Nursing Quarterly, 33*(1), 19–32.

up their part of the bargain, which is to add their "two cents" to the discussion. When individuals do not add their thoughts and comments, other students have nothing to respond to for the discussion. Each participant must take an active role in the conversation for the outcome to be effective.

Technology in the Classroom

Conrad and Donaldson (2004) suggest "lecture is effective for knowledge transmission, but if it is the primary strategy used in the online environment, the course becomes a digital correspondence course with potential problems of learner isolation and high dropout rate" (p. 6). Care must be given to the utilization of technology so that the online delivery is not a digital correspondence course but an exciting, innovative learning environment. The learning outcome must be the "focus of the activity, not the technological tool used to implement the activity" (Conrad & Donaldson, 2004, p. 17). When the tool becomes the key aspect, the content then becomes a secondary aspect of the course, which should not occur. The content needs to be the primary focus.

Connors (2008) states that "in the past 5 years, the number of merging and emerging technologies supported by the Web has increased enormously, making it difficult for faculty members to keep up with the latest advances" (p. 164). With each and every month, new applications of technology are being introduced into the classroom setting. Multiple individuals compare this movement and the resulting expectations for the faculty member as converting from the "sage on the stage" to the "guide on the side." Faculty members are being required to change from delivering the material to facilitating the search for information. Teaching by the "spur of the moment" is not easily applied to the online delivery methodology. Faculty members have to set up the learning environment so that the students are challenged to seek out information and apply that knowledge in multiple processes and situations. Connors (2008) explains this process as "the instructor needs to provide learning experiences that require active learning interaction or collaboration among students, and timely feedback" (p. 167). The formulation of interactive, pedagogically sound opportunities to engage in critical thinking and active decision making is of paramount importance for the success of the learning process. Each of the different technologies must be carefully and effectively incorporated at appropriate times to foster best practices and effective outcomes for the learning environment.

Bleich (2009) suggested that "successful adaptation to Web-based instruction requires competence in modularizing concepts and topics, strategies that engage active learning, and assignments that validate both individual and group attainment of course objectives" (p. 63). Care must be taken by the faculty member to ensure that the adaptation of any course, content, or learning assignment strives to address the expected outcome for the process (see Table 7-4). Over and over, the message is clear that "active learning" is the key for online success. The participants must be stimulated to enthusiastically and dynamically engage with the material presented to assimilate the data into the thinking process. "Being facile with the tools embedded within a technology teaching-learning platform requires work but enlivens learning opportunities and student engagement" (Bleich,

Table 7-4

Recommendations for Successful Online Teaching

- The quality of the instructional delivery for courses needs to be excellent.
- Faculty members should be attuned to the needs of the student cohort.
- Feedback for all courses assignments must be provided to the students in a timely and positive manner.
- Program and course content should be appropriate for the investment required to obtain the degree.
- Activities incorporated within the program of study should reflect innovation, uniqueness, and excite the desire to learn.
- The institution, program, and faculty members must provide timely and appropriate management of requests made by the student cohort.
- Faculty members should provide understandable and comprehensible student assignments within the syllabus.
- Convenient registration should provided for each online course.
- Care must be given to ensure that instructional materials address appropriate course content.
- Programmatic requirements must be unambiguous, realistic, and practical.
- Financial aspects must be equitable and practical.
- Evaluation processes used within the course delivery should be obvious and rational.
- Mechanisms must be in place to help the student access books and other resources needed for courses.

Source: Adapted from Noel-Levitz. (2006). *National online learner priorities report.* Braintree, MA: Author; and Langley, M. E., & Brown, S. T. (2010). Perceptions of the use of reflective learning journals in online graduate nursing education. *Nursing Education Perspective, 31*(1), 12–17.

2009, p. 63). Just to use technology to be able to boast about the tools used does not correlate to effective teaching. Competent and resourceful instruction mandates that learning is accomplished.

Berger, Topp, Davis, Jones, and Stewart (2009) summarized part of the work that was reported in a 2002 study as indicating that participants realized higher grades in online courses; however, the amount of learning was actually related to the enthusiasm and expectations held by the individual student. Online learning is not appropriate for each and every learner. The learner must have the motivation and determination to embrace the learning process. The commitment to the acquisition of knowledge is essential to the success of the individual in the online setting.

Online tools do not increase teaching and learning. The tools are just that—means to an end. Effective use of the tools can potentiate the learning process. Lowenstein and Bradshaw (2004) note, "a tool's effectiveness is determined by the manner in which it is integrated into a course to support the objectives and to create a community of learners" (p. 216). The faculty member's ability to use the tools effectively and efficiently to transfer content is the outcome desired by using a tool.

Since participants can access the tools 24 hours a day, 7 days a week, faculty members should enlighten them as to any limits established for faculty input, such as faculty will not be available 24/7 to respond to student requests. By setting out the limits, frustrations on both sides (students and faculty members) can be reduced. Without the limits, engagement expectations can become overwhelming and unmanageable. Faculty members need to carefully consider "how accessible" they are willing to be given the 24/7 environment of the online delivery mechanism. Adequate communication must take place while ensuring that continuous communication is not required.

According to Kyong-Jee and Bonk (2006), "confusion swells as higher education explores dozens of e-learning technologies (for example, electronic books, simulations, text messaging, podcasting, wikis, blogs), with new ones seeming to emerge each week" (para. 1). With each passing day, new applications of electronic tools are being considered and put to the test within online classes. Some of this utilization has resulted in frustrations. These new applications of the technology tools challenge the education community at a time of budgetary retrenchment and rethinking. The added costs resulting from the acquisition of the new tools and training for the faculty members to be able to use the tools place a burden on the educational community. Care must be given to the best utilization and incorporation of innovative tools into the learning environment so that the goal continues to be the acquisition of learning and knowledge, not the integration of "bells and whistles." Too many bells and whistles without appropriately focusing on the learning can result in bored students who drop courses because the delivery of content is not enriched and engaging.

Jaschik (2009) conducted a meta-analysis of research related to online education. This analysis found that "using technology to give students 'control of their interactions' has a positive effect on student learning" (Jaschik, 2009, para. 8). Within this study, the inclusion of technology tools was determined to be an advantage for engaging the students in a positive manner. The study further determined that "students who took all or part of their instruction online performed better, on average, than those taking the same course through face-to-face instruction" (Jaschik, 2009, para. 2). Although online learning tools seemed to demonstrate a strong correlation for success, the results did not support the superiority of the online delivery application as a method of instruction. "This report correctly recognizes that online learning and blended learning are growing components of higher education and, employed properly, can play a significant role in promoting student learning" (Jaschik, 2009, para. 15). The research included within the meta-analysis sustained the idea of utilizing the methods that best address the content provided and result in successful learning. The linking of instructional methodology and content is the ultimate mechanism for ensuring effectiveness in the learning process.

Evaluation

Bangert and Easterby (2008) affirm that student evaluations of teaching note "that teaching is a complex, multidimensional task that comprises distinct instructional acts" (p. 59S). The process of student evaluation is very complex. Inserting the online delivery technologies adds to the complexity of the process. The evaluation process within online delivery methods must focus on the student materials and not the tools used. Tools are techniques that are outside of the control of the student. Care must be given to ensuring that the assessment of the student is based upon those aspects that are controllable by the student. Included in this consideration is the timing of the assessment. The turning in of assignments has always been compromised by the excuses that students can use. Faculty members need to carefully consider their expectations given the procrastinating student and the potential that Internet access may be compromised. Lateness and/or inability to submit assignments due to the availability of the Internet for whatever reason are areas that each faculty member should consider and address within a course. The availability of Internet access adds to the complexity of the evaluation process. According to Loyola (2010), "the bottom line is that well-designed and well-implemented educational programs determine the effectiveness" (p. 21). Educational institutions must carefully consider the issue of Internet access as well. When students are unable to access the courses in a timely manner for whatever reason, the evaluation and effectiveness of the online program will be impacted. Whether the online delivery platform, Internet portal, or information technology support are the challenge, the quality and functionality of the program will be questioned.

Hanna et al. (2000) stated that as the students partake in an interactive online course, they promptly appreciate that the class is with them all the time. They are compelled to engage with the cohort and react to the materials provided more than is expected in a face-to-face class. The evaluation of the student is based upon this documentation of the engagement within the content of the course. Students cannot sit back and wait—they must actively and appropriately interject their ideas and thoughts into the course to be successful.

Noel-Levitz (2006) states that institutions should identify the issues that are pertinent to students, such as "their interaction with faculty, as well as the service they receive from staff and administrators; the resources provided to students; policies that are in place; and students' overall feelings about the value of the experience" (p. 1). Educational environments that use online methodologies need to understand the experiences both within and outside of the educational context that best contribute to the student's successful completion. Evaluation of the process must address all aspects to guarantee that the student is being heard. Noel-Levitz (2006) suggests that the "research indicates that the greater the fit between expectations and reality, the greater the likelihood for persistence, student success, and stability" (p. 2). Although these aspects are difficult to assess with evaluation tools, mechanisms need to be considered that can address the expectations and realities of the educational experience.

Summary Thoughts

A study reported by Dell, Low, and Wilker (2010) highlights several aspects within online education. This study found that in the United States, over 20% of all higher education students had taken at least one online course in the fall of 2007. This movement of students toward online education continues to encourage faculty members to access and utilize online aspects within the educational process. According to Dell et al. (2010), "online instructors should focus on providing high quality instruction for online learners. Interaction among the learner and with the instructor is important in face-to-face and online formats" (para. 2). This finding further supports the idea that it is the engagement with the students that results in success rather than the methodology. The methodology is used to access the students but is only the means to success. The faculty member's relationship with the students is the foundation for success or lack of success. Dell et al. (2010) determine that for online courses, the "design of the learning environment should include tools to help students with time management, pacing their work load, deadlines that facilitate the completion of their assignments, and appropriate learning strategies" (Conclusion, para. 5). Since the students are not in the classroom or directly accessible, the online delivery must address key aspects to keep the students moving in the correct direction for success. The study further supports the ideas discussed in this chapter when it states "it is important for the instructor to facilitate higher level thinking skills, reflection, and promote problem solving through interactive, problem-based activities" (Dell et al., 2010, Conclusion, para. 5). Faculty members must expect and demand quality interactions and engagement in the learning process. Online courses require the student to strive for excellence in the management of the learning environment. The acquisition of knowledge rests with the student, but is stimulated by the faculty member.

Summary Points

1. During 2004–2008, the number of nurses with an associate's degree (AD) rose from 42.9% to 45.4% (DHHS, 2010).

2. The statistics reflect "among nurses 55 and older, 76,915 intend to leave the nursing profession within 3 years; another 54,539 intend to leave their current nursing job and are unsure if they will remain in nursing afterward" (DHHS, 2010, p. 10).

3. As a result of these dynamics, online educational opportunities are viewed as an innovative, cost-effective approach.

4. Generation X and Millennial cohorts want a learning environment that is accessible, flexible, learner-centered, and meshes with their lifestyle and commitments.

5. Whenever the teacher and the students (learners) are not in the same location, the term *distance education* is applicable.

6. Palloff and Pratt (1999) bring up a very important aspect in regard to distance education when they champion the idea that consideration must be directed toward the development of a community for the participants to facilitate the learning environment.

7. The learners who elect to engage in the educational process from a distance are frequently compelled to do so as a result of time, geographic, financial, or other constraints that restrict their ability to attend traditional classes. The distance learning environment is viewed as convenient, accessible, and flexible.

8. Distance education is viewed as a resourceful and professional alternate for acquiring an advanced degree during economic times that may restrict traveling to a traditional classroom setting.

9. Within the realm of online delivery methodology, any venue or device that allows students and faculty members to engage in the learning process from unique locations can be used.

10. Engaged learning necessitates that the learner becomes directly involved in the entire learning process.

11. Online class participants must engage in the documenting of their nonverbal behavior, whereas in the classroom, learners can simply look around and view the nonverbal communication of their peers. In the face-to-face environment, participants do not have to wait for classmates to engage in documenting their nonverbal feelings.

12. Web-based instruction is any activity/course that is provided via the Internet, also denoted as an online course.

13. The determination of the manner in which the course is delivered should be based on the needs of the student, content to be delivered, mission of the course/program, and expectations of the learning community.

14. The assigned individuals are compelled to be online with the other designated members at the same time for any synchronous activity.
15. Asynchronous activities are viewed as those encounters that are conducted independently of others. Within this process, the learner can address the activity within the course at a time convenient for the individual. Asynchronous activities are done usually within a time period but not needing the direct attention of others.
16. E-books are gaining in attention and utilization within the learning process. E-books are viewed on a computer instead of requiring the purchase of hard copies or printed textbooks.
17. Chickering and Gamson (1987) stated that effective management of the undergraduate educational experience required the encouraging of connection concerning students and faculty, cultivating teamwork among students, advancing vigorous learning, providing timely feedback, articulating quality expectations, and recognizing distinct techniques of learning; such concerns are similar in an online environment.
18. Since students are not sitting in the room with their colleagues and the faculty member, attention to methods for allowing the individuals within the course to connect as a learning community is of paramount importance.
19. Superficial scrutiny of the material presented does not allow for the full acquisition of the content to be assimilated from the course.
20. Online delivery of the educational experience places a lot of responsibility squarely on the learner.
21. Care must be given to the utilization of technology so that the online delivery is not a digital correspondence course but an exciting, innovative learning environment.
22. Over and over, the message is clear that "active learning" is the key for online success. The participants must be stimulated to enthusiastically and dynamically engage with the material presented to assimilate the data into the thinking process. Just to use technology to be able to boast about the tools used does not correlate to effective teaching.
23. Online learning is not appropriate for each and every learner.
24. New applications of technology tools challenge the education community at a time of budgetary retrenchment and rethinking. The added cost resulting from the acquisition of the new tools and training for the faculty members to be able to use the tools places a burden on the educational community.
25. Care must be given to ensure that the assessment of students is based on aspects that are controlled by the student.
26. The availability of Internet access adds to the complexity of the evaluation process.
27. When students are unable to access the courses in a timely manner for whatever reason, the evaluation and effectiveness of the online program will be impacted.

Tips for Nurse Educators to Use

1. The learners who elect to engage in the educational process from a distance are frequently compelled to do so as a result of time, geographic, financial, or other constraints that restrict their ability to attend traditional classes.

2. While the computer and Internet tend to be the most frequently utilized aspects for online delivery, other devices are being incorporated as technology grows and develops.

3. Within the online community, the participants can remain neutral if desired. If a peer does not engage, the primary indication that a problem is developing may only be decreased communication by that individual.

4. Web-based instruction requires active learning and engagement in the learning process by the individual student.

5. Within asynchronous activities, the learner can address the activity within the course at a time convenient for the individual. Asynchronous activities are done usually within a time period but not needing the direct attention of others.

6. E-books allow for quick turnaround when updates are needed. Since the books are accessed via the computer or iPod device, a question can be quickly researched to determine up-to-date information when making critical decisions.

7. Rules/recommendations for online communication, called netiquette, include the use of capital letters, proper use of the computer, management of emails, and so forth.

8. Taking the time to plan how to unite the different members in the course cohort is a critical foundation for the development of discussion and interactions. Since the individuals don't have the advantage of sitting in a room together, the development of a comfort level with the different individuals must take place through the use of communication skills.

9. Learning objectives are the underpinning for the educational experience; thus, each and every activity to be incorporated into a course needs to be scrutinized to determine its functionality.

10. To be effective, the teacher should determine the results expected from the engagement in the learning process.

11. The process of summarizing within an online course mandates that the participant scrutinize and dissect the content to a moderately multifaceted and meaningful degree.

12. Since a faculty member is not directly with the students, the need for recognition and immediacy is increased. Faculty members need to contemplate when and how to provide recognition and encouragement that is timely and directed.

13. Online sessions move rapidly and require each member of the cohort to be self-directed and engaged.

14. When the technological tools become the key aspect, the content then becomes a secondary aspect of the course, which should not occur.

15. Faculty members within an online delivery process are charged with facilitating the search for the information, not the delivery of the material.

16. Faculty members have to set up the learning environment so that the students are challenged to seek out information and apply that knowledge in multiple processes and situations.

17. Care must be taken by the faculty member to ensure that the online adaptation of any course, content, or learning assignment strives to address the expected outcome for the process.

18. Lateness and/or inability to submit assignments due to the availability of the Internet for whatever reason are areas that each faculty member should consider and address within a course.

19. Students cannot sit back and wait—they must actively and appropriately interject their ideas and thoughts into the course to be successful.

20. The faculty member's relationship with students is the foundation for success or lack of success.

21. Since the students are not in the classroom or directly accessible, the online delivery must address key aspects to keep the students moving in the correct direction for success.

References

Bangert, A. W., & Easterby, L. (2008). Designing and delivering effective online nursing courses with the evolve electronic classroom. CIN: Computer, Informatic, Nursing, 26(2), 99–105.

Bastable, S. B. (2003). Nurse as educator: Principles of teaching and learning for nursing practice (2nd ed.). Sudbury, MA: Jones and Bartlett Publishers.

Berger, J., Topp, R., Davis, L., Jones, J., & Stewart, L. (2009, May/June). Comparison of web-based and face-to-face training concerning patient education within a hospital system. Journal for Nurses in Staff Development, 127–132.

Bleich, M. F. (2009). Technology: An imperative for teaching in the age of digital natives. Journal of Nursing Education, 48(2), 63.

Chickering, A. W., & Gamson, Z. F. (1987, March). Seven principles for good practice in undergraduate education. The American Association for Higher Education Bulletin.

Connors, H. R. (2008). Beyond the classroom: Considering distance education approaches. In B. K. Penn (Ed.), Mastering the teaching role: A guide for nurse educator (pp. 163–175). Philadelphia, PA: F.A. Davis.

Conrad, R., & Donaldson, J. A. (2004) Engaging the online learner: Activities and resources for creative instruction. San Francisco, CA: Jossey-Bass Publishers.

Dell, C. A., Low, C., & Wilker, J. F. (2010). Comparing student achievement in online and face-to-face class formats. Journal of Online Learning and Teaching, 6(1). Retrieved May 14, 2010, from http://jolt.merlot.org/vol6no1/dell_0310.htm

Dorin, M. D. (2009, February). Cyber-instructor? Consider becoming an online educator. Nursing Management, 34–37.

Draves, W. A. (2000). Teaching online. River Falls, WI: LERN books.

Hanna, D. E., Glowacki-Dudka, M., & Conceicao-Runlee, S. (2000). 147 practical tips for teaching online groups: Essentials of web-based education. Madison, WI: Atwood Publishing.

Jaschik, S. (2009). The evidence on online education. Retrieved April 5, 2010, from http://www.insidehighered.com/layout/set/print/news/2009/29/online

Kyong-Jee, K., & Bonk, C. J. (2006). The future of online teaching and learning in higher education: The survey says . . . EDUCAUSE Quarterly, 29(4). Retrieved May 14, 2010, from http://www.educause.edu/node/157426.?time=1291863108

Leski, J. (2009). Nursing students and faculty perceptions of computer-based instruction at a 2-year college. Journal of Nursing Education, 48(2), 91–95.

Lowenstein, A. J., & Bradshaw, M. J. (2004). Fuszard's innovative teaching strategies in nursing (3rd ed.). Sudbury, MA: Jones and Bartlett Publishers.

Loyola, S. (2010). Evidence-based teaching guidelines: Transforming knowledge into practice for better outcomes in healthcare. Critical Care Nursing Quarterly, 33(1), 19–32.

Noel-Levitz. (2006). National online learner priorities report. Braintree, MA: Author.

Palloff, R. M., & Pratt, K. (1999). Building learning communities in cyberspace: Effective strategies for the online classroom. San Francisco, CA: Jossey-Bass Publishers.

Tri-Council for Nursing. (2010). Educational advancement of registered nurses: A consensus position. Washington, DC: Author.

U.S. Department of Health and Human Services, Health Resources and Services Administration. (2010). The registered nurse population: Initial findings from the 2008 *national sample survey of registered nurses.* Washington, DC: U.S. Department of Health and Human Services, Health Resources and Services Administration.

Williams, M. G., & Dittmer, A. (2009). Textbooks on tap: Using electronic books housed in handheld devices in nursing clinical courses. *Nursing Education Perspectives, 30*(4), 220–225.

Web Links

For information related to self-assessment in distance learning, visit http://elearning
.kumc.edu/about.html#skill session and http://ittraining.iu.edu/workshops/
deguide/de_student_primer.pdf.

View the Second Life home page at http://secondlife.com/whatis.

See Clayton R. Wright's article on criteria for evaluating the quality of online courses
at http://elearning.typepad.com/thelearnedman/ID/evaluatingcourses.pdf.

The Quality Matters Rubric Standards, 2008–2010 edition with Assigned Point Values, is available at http://qminstitute.org/home/Public%20Library/About%
20QM/RubricStandards2008-2010.pdf.

For more information on netiquette rules, visit www.albion.com/netiquette/
corerules.html and www.kassj.com/netiquette/netiquette.html.

Multiple Choice Questions

1. Generation X and the Millennial generation expect a learning process that is:
   A. flexible, teacher-centered, and open to lifestyles.
   B. flexible, learner-centered, and committed to different lifestyles.
   C. rigid, learner-centered, and committed to specific learning processes.
   D. rigid, teacher-centered, and committed to different lifestyles.

   Rationale:

   Generation X and Millennial cohorts want a learning environment that is accessible, flexible, learner-centered, and meshes with their lifestyle and commitments.

2. Examples of distance learning opportunities include:
   A. online courses, correspondence courses, and independent studies.
   B. online courses, videoconferencing, and regular courses.
   C. correspondence courses only.
   D. online courses only.

   Rationale:

   Bastable (2003) list examples of distance learning as online courses, correspondence courses, independent study, and videoconferencing. Whenever the teacher and the students (learners) are not in the same location, this term is applicable.

3. Some of the reasons that students elect to participate in distance education opportunities are:
   A. time, geographic, and financial liberties.
   B. convenience, accessibility, and rigidity.
   C. time restrictions, flexibility, and geographic considerations.
   D. commitment to excellence, rigidity, and structure.

   Rationale:

   The learners who elect to engage in the educational process from a distance are frequently compelled to do it as a result of time, geographic, financial, or other constraints that restrict their ability to attend traditional classes. The distance learning environment is viewed as convenient, accessible, and flexible.

4. Engaged learning requires the learner to:
   A. be a passive learner.
   B. follow the lead of the faculty member.
   C. engage as needed.
   D. become directly involved in the learning process.

Rationale:

According to Conrad and Donaldson (2004), "engaged learning is focused on the learner, whose role is integral to the generation of new knowledge" (p. 5). Engaged learning necessitates that the learner become directly involved in the entire learning process. The learner is an active participant in the process. Lowenstein and Bradshaw (2004) postulate that "participation in any form of distance learning requires students to be self-directed and able to function in an environment with limited faculty feedback and lacking face-to-face interaction" (p. 213). Students who engage in distance learning opportunities must understand that the responsibility for learning falls upon them, as they don't have the classroom to use for passive learning.

5. Synchronous activities are those activities within an online course that require:
   A. **all members of the cohort to be online at the same time**.
   B. a few members of the cohort to be online at the same time.
   C. engagement in the activity at a time conducive for the participant.
   D. engagement in the activity at the same time by the cohort only.

Rationale:

Synchronous activities are those planned activities where all of the members are expected to be online and/or connected at the same time.

6. Asynchronous activities within an online course are those that require activities to be posted:
   A. at a time convenient for the faculty member.
   B. at a time convenient for the cohort.
   C. **at a time convenient for the learner**.
   D. all at the same time.

Rationale:

Asynchronous activities are viewed as those encounters that are conducted independently of others. Within this process, the learner can address the activity within the course at a time convenient for the individual. Asynchronous activities are done usually within a time period but not needing the direct attention of others.

7. Topics that are harder to address via a computer-based delivery methodology are those that
   A. are stand-alone topics.
   B. **require hands-on management**.
   C. need faculty in attendance.
   D. are complex.

Rationale:

Computer-based instruction is functional for some areas but inappropriate for other areas. Those topics that require hands-on management pose difficulty when considered for presentation via a computer-based delivery methodology.

8.   Bundled e-book packages have the advantage of:

   A.   allowing quick turnaround when updates are needed.
   B.   requiring students to be technological savvy.
   C.   restricting access to the package when not at school.
   D.   allowing anyone to change the package as needed to update it.

Rationale:

E-books are gaining in attention and utilization within the learning process. E-books are viewed on a computer instead of requiring the purchasing of hard copies or printed textbooks. The computer-based delivery of the books allows for quick turnaround when updates are needed.

9.   Netiquette rules and recommendations are considered as methods for ensuring:

   A.   assertive management of the online communication.
   B.   passive engagement with fellow students.
   C.   civilized interactions with individuals on the web.
   D.   control within a classroom setting.

Rationale:

Netiquette rules and recommendations include the use of capital letters, proper use of the computer, management of emails, and so forth. Netiquette is viewed as the behaviors that reflect being civilized on the computer.

10.   To ensure connection between faculty members and students, the educational experience should:

   A.   discourage vigorous learning as it will disrupt the learning process.
   B.   recognize specific techniques of learning to facilitate the process.
   C.   articulate the expectations for individual work, not team activities, within the process.
   D.   hold feedback until the end of the process to allow the student to be creative.

Rationale:

Chickering and Gamson (1987) state that effective management of the undergraduate educational experience required the encouraging of connection concerning students and faculty, cultivating teamwork among students, advancing vigorous learning, providing timely feedback, articulating quality expectations, and recognizing distinct techniques of learning. Online learning environments must include these aspects as well.

11. Characteristics that need to be evidenced when attempting to engage and facilitate online courses are:
   A. directness, truthfulness, rigidity, and disregard.
   B. disrespect, relevance, openness, and empowerment.
   C. duplicity, sensitivity, openness, and empowerment.
   D. honesty, responsiveness, openness, and empowerment.

Rationale:

According to Palloff and Pratt (1999), "the keys to the creation of a learning community and successful facilitation online are simple—honesty, responsiveness, relevance, respect, openness, and empowerment" (p. 20). Taking the time to plan how to unite the different members in the course cohort is a critical piece foundational for the development of discussion and interactions.

12. Online delivery does not have the advantage of the classroom as a method for developing the comfort levels within the cohort. What method is paramount for use within the online delivery mechanisms for establishing a comfort level with the members of the class?
   A. Multiple assignments
   B. Use of hands-on assignments
   C. Use of communication skills
   D. Assignments that require ongoing communication

Rationale:

Taking the time to plan how to unite the different members in the course cohort is a critical foundation for the development of discussion and interactions. Since the individuals don't have the advantage of sitting in a room together, the development of a comfort level with the different individuals must be done through the use of communication skills.

13. Engagement of the learner in the educational process necessitates that the faculty member find ways to encourage
   A. networking for the members of the class.
   B. individualization of the learning process.
   C. independence from the other members of the class.
   D. collaboration with the faculty member.

Rationale:

The faculty member must establish multiple venues for granting access to peers and faculty. Since the delivery is online and not face-to-face, every opportunity for engaging the participants (students and faculty) must be provided and encouraged. The opportunities to engage with peers and the faculty are the aspect that connects the individuals together in the learning process and aids in the networking for the members of the cohort involved in the online sessions.

14. The key focus for any online course should be the:

    A. process.
    B. technological tools.
    C. content.
    D. individuals in the course.

Rationale:

When technological tools become the key aspect, the content then becomes a secondary aspect of the course, which should not occur. The content needs to be the primary focus.

15. The design of the learning environment for an online course should address:

    A. time management, workload pace, deadlines, and appropriate learning strategies.
    B. scheduling of outside assignments, teaching strategies, and workload.
    C. scheduling of all aspects of the student's time and pacing of outside endeavors.
    D. time management, self-confidence, and building of respect.

Rationale:

Dell et al. (2010) determine that for online courses, the "design of the learning environment should include tools to help students with time management, pacing their work load, deadlines that facilitate the completion of their assignments, and appropriate learning strategies" (Conclusion, para. 5). Since the students are not in the classroom or directly accessible, the online delivery must address key aspects to keep the students moving in the correct direction for success. The study further supports the ideas discussed in this chapter when it states "it is important for the instructor to facilitate higher level thinking skills, reflection, and promote problem solving through interactive, problem-based activities" (Dell et al., 2010, Conclusion, para. 5).

Discussion Questions

1. In an online delivery format, what type of strategies would a faculty member need to consider to ensure that the learning environment was at an optimum level for the students?

2. From the list of suggestions provided concerning planning and conducting online courses, select three to four of the suggestions and discuss how each could be used in improving a course currently taught or being prepared for teaching.

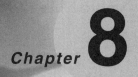

Chapter **8**

Clinical Educational Experiences

Joyce Miller and Carol Boswell

Chapter Objectives

At the conclusion of this chapter, the learner will be able to:

1. Discuss the differences and similarities between clinical judgment, clinical reasoning, and clinical decision making.
2. Explain the uses of high-fidelity simulation, low-fidelity simulation, and static manikins.
3. Examine the evidence related to clinical simulation.
4. Discuss methodologies educators, preceptors, and coaches can use to incorporate evidence-based activities in clinical settings.
5. Identify a variety of venues for student evaluations in the clinical setting from the perspective of educator, preceptor, or coach.

Key Terms

➤ Clinical decision making

➤ Clinical judgment

➤ Clinical reasoning

➤ Coaching

➤ Cognitive knowledge acquisition

➤ Debriefing

➤ Experiential learning

➤ High-fidelity simulation

➤ Low-fidelity simulation

➤ Moderate-fidelity simulation

➤ Preceptors

➤ Self-confidence

➤ Self-efficacy

➤ Static manikin

Introduction

As nursing education moves forward into the next decade, the concepts of evidence-based teaching and clinical competency that can be acquired using simulation and other resources have taken on new meaning and importance. The acknowledgement of innovative opportunities to bring the skills and applications to the students must be embraced and embedded into the educational process as we advance the profession of nursing. New and innovative means of providing clinical experiences have been researched to manage the growing problem confronting many schools of nursing across the country. Adams and Valiga (2009) submit that the challenge within the current healthcare environment is to provide students with a full and efficient variety of clinical learning opportunities while dealing with the restrictions encountered by fewer clinical resources. As the challenge of fewer clinical settings resulting in increasing problems when trying to locate clinical sites becomes a reality, the concept of simulation becomes progressively more imperative within the educational environment (Adams & Valiga, 2009; Bambino, Washburn, & Perkins, 2009; Letvak, 2008). This chapter examines the provision of clinical learning opportunities. With the number of schools proliferating due to the current and anticipated future nursing workforce shortage, clinical placements are becoming scarce. As a result, many schools and state boards of nursing are considering more time spent in clinical simulation as an option.

Letvak (2008) suggests that an ideal clinical setting is one that presents encounters that are applicable, pertinent, and timely for the content being presented within the courses and that offer opportunities to reinforce and practice the skills already acquired. So no matter in what location the clinical experience is provided or what resources are used, the ultimate criterion for the learning process is the acquisition of skills in a timely manner while also supporting and confirming skills already learned.

Jeffries (2008) defines evidence-based teaching as "using 'best evidence' to select, develop, and implement educational strategies and conducting research to further define educational practice" (slide 14). For this text, evidence-based teaching (EBT) is a dynamic, holistic system using educational principles validated by evidence to support, maintain, and promote a new level of knowledge for a learner in a variety of settings. Evidence-based teaching must strive to locate the best evidence instead of depending on the patterns used over the decades. Jeffries (2008) goes on to list three reasons why EBT is important: (1) integrating pedagogical research results helps in the development of a foundational body of knowledge related to health-care education, (2) utilizing teaching strategies that have been identi-fied by evidence allows for stability within learning outcomes, and (3) incorporating evidence-based instructional tactics provides a means for replication, refinement, and establishment of "best prac-tices." These three motivations for moving toward EBT provide a foundation for the effective incorporation of evidence and the estab-lishment of excellence within nursing education. Adams and Valiga (2009) stated that "Excellence means striving to be the very best you can be in everything you do—not because some . . . 'authority' fig-ure [demands it], but because you can't imagine functioning in any other way. It means setting high standards for yourself and the groups in which you are involved, holding yourself to those standards despite challenges or pressures to reduce or lower them, and not being satis-fied with anything less than the very best" (p. 3). Within each and every endeavor in the educational process, excellence should be and is the goal for the development of an effective nursing profession.

Instructional Settings

Clinical experiences are a mainstay within nursing educational activi-ties. Since nursing is viewed to be both an art and a science, the "hands-on" aspect is highly valued within all nursing programs. Clini-cal experiences allow the practical application of the information covered during the didactic aspects of the program. Clinical sites can include acute care agencies, secondary schools, day cares, senior cen-ters, home health agencies, hospice settings, mobile clinics, physician and/or nurse practitioner managed clinics, industrial health clinics, and community agencies. By using the material provided with actual and/or simulated clients, students are better able to understand and effectively use the information as they work to apply safe nursing care. The instructional settings used for these clinical experiences can be a variety of agencies and resources. Any location where individuals are seen and encountered can be a potential clinical site. Clinical experi-ences are really the interactions with people, not the physical settings where these might happen. As a result, faculty members have to be constantly open to new and innovative locations that may meet the course needs. The basic driving force related to clinical experiences is the course objectives. The course objectives are those concepts and skills that need to be attained during a given clinical engagement.

Faculty members within selected courses need to be persistently searching for appropriate agencies and settings where the objectives for that course can be attained.

As faculty members identify potential clinical agencies, the nursing program has the responsibility for establishing a relationship with the designated group. According to Misener (2008), this responsibility must be shared by faculty, the dean's office, and the central administration for locating clinical facilities. Frequently, the actual clinical contract or affiliation agreement is developed and maintained through the dean's office and the central administration for the clinical agreements. The central administration holds the accountability for ensuring that any contract/agreement is in compliance with all university rules and regulations. The dean assumes the responsibility for assuring that the areas covered in the contract/agreements are complied with for the partnership. This relationship that is formed needs to be symbiotic, synergistic, and must address the mission of the university and the clinical agency. The partnerships should always reflect a "win-win" situation for the groups involved in the joint venture. The faculty members hold the accountability for maintaining the different aspects related to a clinical association. Both the university and the agency are expected to preserve an infrastructure that supports the aspects covered by the agreement. One key aspect that is paramount to the successful management of clinical affiliations is communication. All parties involved in the educational process must be committed to maintaining and augmenting the partnership as the clinical experiences move forward. It takes everyone's involvement and commitment to effectively communicate needs, successes, and barriers.

According to Letvak (2008), factors that are important within the selection and management of clinical sites are:

- Course objectives
- Consistency between the agency's and school of nursing's philosophy
- Maintenance of a high standard of care
- Reasonability of commute distance for students
- Provision of adequate parking and safety when students are traveling between parking lot and agency
- Availability of food service or storage for students to bring their own food
- Accessibility to conference or meeting space
- Commitment and positive interactions by agency staff with students

With the changing environment of health care and academia, other areas that also need to be considered when selecting clinical experiences are directly related to the type of clinical experiences needed.

Computer access is one area that is gaining in importance. Another area for consideration is the availability of current textbooks and resources for the students to use as they endeavor to provide safe and effective health care to the clients.

Simulation

One such way to provide and support the acquisition of clinical skills and competency is the use of simulation, which has taken on new importance with the restrictions placed on clinical resources. As increasing enrollments, nursing shortages, agency accreditation requirements, and current scares within the media about problems within the healthcare arena place a toll on healthcare agencies, clinical resources are becoming harder and harder to attain. Jeffries (2009) asserts that "clinical simulation offers students rich, authentic clinical experiences in a safe, nonthreatening environment" (p. 71). Through the use of simulation, students are provided the opportunities to try out new skills prior to performing them on real patients (Bambino et al., 2009; Cato, Lasater, & Peeples, 2009; Jeffries, 2009; Smith & Roehrs, 2009). With the complexities of the inpatient population, simulation activities allow the students to acquire knowledge with situations prior to being placed in that setting. By having the opportunities to work through problems with the use of a device, students and faculty members can provide educational materials, evaluate the different options, and incorporate research while in a safe, nonthreatening environment.

Let's clarify some words and concepts frequently used within the world of simulation. The first term that needs to be considered is **experiential learning**. Experiential learning implies that the learning is done by a person or through a program/activity structured by others (Neill, 2005). Within this form of learning, the emphasis is placed on active participation by all members involved (Thomas Dreifuerst, 2009). Within the context of the different generational cohorts discussed in earlier chapters, experiential learning is seen as a valuable way to engage them and to incorporate the use of group/cohort work. As individuals take an active part in the learning process, genuine, meaningful, and long-lasting learning occurs.

Two additional terms to become familiar with are **self-efficacy** and **self-confidence**. Van Wagner (n.d.) postulates that self-efficacy is directly related to Bandura's work on social cognitive theory. Self-efficacy is viewed as an individual's conviction in his or her capacity to thrive in a given situation. Self-confidence goes along the same lines. It is understood to be a certainty in the capacity, credibility, or dependability of a person. As a person develops self-efficacy and self-confidence, he or she becomes adept at confronting challenges successfully, seeking learning opportunities, developing commitment to the learning process, and recovering promptly from obstacles and disappointments. Successful management of simulation activities is viewed as a means to improve self-efficacy within the student. As a result, the student is then better able to move forward successfully within the educational environment.

According to Thomas Dreifuerst (2009), "mastery of critical thinking, clinical decision making, and clinical judgment is a milestone of professional development as a nurse moves from being a novice to becoming an expert clinician" (p. 109). Critical thinking was discussed and defined in Chapter 1 of this textbook. **Clinical decision making** works with critical thinking through the use of nursing knowledge, proficiency, and viewpoints to ascertain an appropriate action and/or response. **Clinical reasoning** then takes the critical thinking and clinical decision making together with additional cognitive elements to see beyond the obvious solutions to innovative management of the clinical situation. **Clinical judgment** is established by identification of the dynamic transitions by individuals across time as ·they react to health concerns and associated treatment (Benner, 1984). Each of these clinical aspects is somewhat of a staircase to higher levels of utilization within the clinical setting. As individuals gain confidence, the information used within the decision-making process is increased, thus allowing for more complex management of the client situation. A final aspect within this process is **cognitive knowledge acquisition**. Cognitive learning is understood to incorporate listening to, watching, touching, and experiencing the world around us (ThinkQuest Team, n.d.). As our brains manipulate the physical objects and events encountered, the information is processed and formulated into retrieval memories. Cognitive knowledge acquisition is considered to be an active process of learning that engages and stimulates the individual to view items from many different perspectives instead of as one-dimensional objects.

Let's move to the differences within the process of simulation. Some of the terms used are *static manikin, low-fidelity simulation, moderate-fidelity simulation,* and *high-fidelity simulation.* **Static manikins** are those partial task trainers that are used to practice specific skills, such as ear or prostate manikins (Simulation Innovation and Resource Center, n.d.). Static manikins can be at either the low-fidelity or moderate-fidelity level. **Low-fidelity simulation** (LFS) experiences are those opportunities for the students to engage in case studies, role playing, or group activities that are specific to a narrow skill process. Static manikins at this level would be restricted to one narrow task practice, such as the ear or prostate manikins. According to Adams and Valiga (2009), "high fidelity and medium [moderate] fidelity simulators are life-like mannequins, referred to as human patient simulators that are programmed to mimic the responses of a human being" (p. 100). **Moderate-fidelity simulation** (MFS) includes those models that are two-dimensional in their focus on the experience being learned, such as IV arms. This level does encourage problem solving within the management of the manikin case study. Spunt and Covington (2008) advocate that "high-fidelity simulation offers the most realistic clinical experience possible, short of caring for a real patient, and may involve advanced equipment that interacts with the learner" (p. 234). With **high-fidelity simulation** (HFS), the case presentations can be complicated and in-depth; Harvey simulators are an example. Dillon, Noble, and Kaplan (2009) relate that the HFS process provides incomparable opportunities that allow the students to practice skills within a safe and controlled environment. They also recommend HFS activities because they allow the presentation of clinical experiences that may not be as frequently encountered within the healthcare setting. Spunt and Covington (2008) sum up the use of simulators as enabling "the student to experience simple or complex, stable or unpredictable clinical situations before encountering real ones in the clinical setting" (p. 234). Because the situation is controlled by the faculty members involved, the depth of the clinical situation with the incorporation of key knowledge points can be managed and addressed during the simulation experience prior to the student confronting the aspects within a real-world setting. Depending on the clinical opportunities available at different sites, some skills and tasks may not be readily available for all of the students to manage. The simulation process is well positioned to address these skills and tasks for the entire cohort.

An understanding of each of these terms is paramount for synthesizing the evidence related to simulation. Each of these different aspects is directly related to the effective utilization of this teaching strategy within the clinical arena. Adams and Valiga (2009) stated that simulation and simulated case scenarios are an effective means for appraising and examining clinical skills, critical thinking, and clinical judgments within the context of re-creating the healthcare needs from a client's viewpoint. Tagliareni (2009) stated that "throughout our history, nurse educators have used simulation to teach basic skills, to promote mastery of tasks in the clinical lab, and to replicate practice situation" (p. 69). Simulation has become the hope for the future within nursing education. With the many challenges confronting nursing education and the call to change the way that nursing is being taught, simulation is viewed as a lifeline that is appropriate for addressing these concerns and challenges. Smith (2009) relates that HFS activities within skills labs are predominantly used to ensure the learning of skills and tasks. Smith (2009) goes on to say that the use of HFS activities within a simulated clinical setting incorporates the solving of problems, encourages teamwork, facilitates a better understanding of complex disease problems, and augments decision making and critical thinking. At this point, let's look at what a few of the experts say about simulation. The concepts put forth by the experts are based on research evidence and practical application evidence.

Spunt and Covington (2008) provide a well-rounded look at the ideas included within clinical simulation activities. One of the advantages of the use of this teaching strategy is that the learner must be self-directed because the environment is interactive. The learner is called on to engage and advance the scenario at a speed reflective of individual needs and knowledge. Another advantage for the use of simulation is the opportunity for faculty members to be able to provide missing experiences that have not been provided within the actual clinical setting or that can't be done by all of the members of the cohort. By using the clinical simulation option, those clinical scenarios can be provided to each member of the cohort without having to locate the experience within the authentic clinical setting. Thus, the students can benefit from the learning without having to be stressed to locate a patient with that disease or equipment. As has already been discussed, clinical simulation provides opportunities for the students to apply their didactic knowledge and problem-solving skills, critical thinking abilities, and time management skills. Because the clinical simulation activities allow time for the students to think about time management and aspects of care, skills in managing time effectively in the busy world of health care and appropriate delegation can be contemplated and determined in a safe environment. Spunt and Covington (2008) continue to acknowledge that due to the safe environment provided by the clinical simulation setting, the students learn faster because they do not perceive personal threats and barriers. From the evidence, clinical simulations are valued from the first undergraduate semester through to the graduate program with specialized clinical applications and all the way to the doctoral research programs. Simulations allow the faculty members to adjust variations based upon the current healthcare arena and the learning needs of the participants. As new and innovative changes are encountered in the workplace, changes can be made to the scenarios to address these changes. Also, as political changes occur, such as in national healthcare policy, these aspects can be incorporated into the scenario to allow for the currency of the educational process. Spunt and Covington (2008) acknowledge the positive benefit of the clinical simulation related to reflective opportunities. Students and faculty members can reflect on the processes utilized within the scenarios to advance the profession of nursing.

Smith and Roehrs (2009) provide several key thoughts related to the evidence associated with the use of clinical situations. Historically, nursing education has employed a variety of simulation activities for clinical experiences, involving static manikins, task trainers, case studies, and role playing. Although these types of activities offer advantages depending on the objectives and cost constraints of the institution, "they do not provide students with a realistic context for performing nursing skills or the opportunity to learn to perform a skill while interacting with a patient" (Smith & Roehrs, 2009, p. 74). The use of HFS provides these extra benefits within a simulation activity. For a clinical simulation to be effective, the evidence shows that the designing of the scenario should embrace five related aspects:

- clear objectives and information;
- support during the simulation;
- a suitable problem to solve;
- time for guided reflection/feedback; and
- fidelity or realism of the experience.

The research done by Smith and Roehrs (2009) suggests "that having clear objectives and an appropriate problem to solve requires special consideration by nurse education when designing an HFS experience" (p. 77). Faculty members must embrace the idea that clinical simulations require the pre-session work of planning and management of the learning expectations. Each scenario and engagement should be carefully deliberated to identify and clarify the objectives and problems to be confronted within the scenario. Though some areas of the clinical process will be unique based upon the decisions made by the students, the foundational expectations for the learning session must be carefully and thoroughly planned and incorporated into the learning packet for the session.

Another source of evidence related to clinical simulations is provided by Bambino et al. (2009). They identified three themes related to areas that were supported and addressed via this teaching strategy. The initial theme related to communication, both verbal and nonverbal. "Participants [in the study] indicated that they learned the importance of communicating with significant others as well as the patient" (Bambino et al., 2009, p. 81). The second premise was associated with the confidence gained in the areas of psychomotor skills and patient interactions. Through the use of clinical simulation activities, students thought they gained confidence by "letting them know what to expect and giving them experiences in working through assessments and problem solving" (Bambino et al., 2009, p. 81). The final idea was associated with clinical judgment. The importance of prioritizing assessment skills, determining when and how to intervene, and identifying aspects concerning abnormal physical assessment findings were facets of clinical judgment that were thought to be improved from engaging in these clinical scenarios. The work done by Bambino et al. (2009) also identified that the aspect within clinical skills that is missing in traditional skill lab experiences is the context of the process. Clinical simulation allows for an improved addressing of the context of the material, skills, and goals for the session. The complexities of context within a clinical simulation activity require the students to be able to reprioritize and modify rules and situations based upon the needs of the client and the healthcare assessments. Bambino et al. (2009) concluded that "simulation can introduce novice students to the process of being able to perceive characteristics and aspects of patient care situations that may alter the manner in which nursing care is provided" (p. 79). By utilizing the clinical simulation process, students' self efficacy and self-confidence were strengthened. Students were found to be able to work through patient encounters with increasing complexities of patient care to provide nursing care that was safe, resulting in reduced errors in clinical judgment and fewer potential harmful situations for living clients.

Further evidence is provided by Hoadley (2009) for the use of clinical simulation. It is recommended that "with the use of HFS, nurses can improve skill versatility and increase self-confidence" (p. 95). This development of self-confidence is an outcome of amplified internalization of the content provided and improved satisfaction with the learning environment. A final aspect supported by Hoadley (2009) is that "the incorporation of experiential learning and reflection/debriefing enhances knowledge by developing one or both of the following behaviors: retention and transferences" (p. 92). This research study further supports that idea that the "hands-on" experiences created by clinical simulation opportunities allow students to better grasp the complexity of nursing care provision. Students emerge with confidence in being able to direct the complex care of clients after having been exposed to these types of client situations in the less threatening environment of clinical simulation.

The research work completed by Elfrink, Nininger, Rohig, and Lee (2009) provides additional evidence-based teaching considerations. From the work done by Elfrink et al. (2009), "best practices for simulation design in nursing education incorporate learner support in the form of hints, cues, or direction, offered before, during and after simulation experiences" (p. 83). Faculty members must be attentive to the use of hints, cues, and direction. These aspects must be inserted habitually within the scenario, not as a one-time-only occurrence. As faculty members consider the generational aspects of learners, this point becomes even more important. By providing the hints, cues, and directions throughout the scenario, the generational cohort can see the expertise held by the faculty members and develop respect for the knowledge base and authority residing within the faculty members. The work of Elfrink et al. (2009) produced two aspects that need to be carefully considered. Within this study, students found the use of videotaping of the simulation experience to be very stressful and unproductive. The students related that they were distracted by the worry related to the taping. Faculty members viewed the videotape as helpful for the debriefing sessions. Students, on the other hand, found the use of the videotape during the debriefing sessions to be negative. Another concern that they raised was the negativity resulting from having to repeat the simulation. Repeating the same simulation was seen as more busywork than productive learning time. From this study, the students suggested that the content and management of the debriefing session be strengthened instead of repeating any simulation experience, and that videotapes not be used to review the experience. A positive aspect that resulted from this research study was the recommendation of using planning sessions. "A large number of students felt that a planning session following the patient hand-off and report would be a productive step toward lessening anxiety, placing a particular student 'on the spot' and facilitating 'where to start'" (Elfrink et al., 2009, p. 85). This idea of planning sessions concurs with the generational aspects related to Generation X that support group engagement. It allows the group to work through the anticipated scenario to be prepared for what is expected. The student group would still need to deal with the unexpected complexities that emerge during the scenario. The preplanning allows for teamwork and an interactive, collaborative process. Elfrink et al. (2009) concluded that "promoting an environment of collaborative learning has the potential to increase ownership in the entire simulation experience" (p. 86). This evidence strongly supports and upholds the evidence noted about the strengths and challenges presented by the different generational cohorts. The incorporation of teamwork and collaboration is directly supportive of the characteristics within these different generational groups.

Dillon et al. (2009) provide additional evidence related to the appropriateness of clinical simulation by noting that "receiving immediate feedback, without the possibility of causing patient harm, allows students to develop a repertoire of possible solutions" (p. 87). Feedback without the threat of penalty supports the characteristics seen within the generational cohorts. As an experiential learning technique and strategy, simulation promotes the cohort to associate the applicable concepts, employ suitable theories in clinical practice, and determine satisfactory clinical decisions. From the work done by this team of researchers, simulation was found to endorse the skills of communication, teamwork, delegation, priority setting, and leadership.

The work done by Cato et al. (2009) turns the research toward the aspect of **debriefing** within the clinical simulation process. The evidence found within this study further supported the idea that the clinical simulation process was instrumental in developing the students' clinical judgment and critical thinking skills. The process of the clinical simulation endeavor frequently takes the path of one group interacting directly in the scenario while another group serves as reviewers of the process. Following the completion of the scenario, the entire group comes together for a debriefing process. Cato et al. (2009) state that the "debriefing that follows each scenario focuses on the team's care of the patient, including safe practice, priority setting, continuous assessment, communication, resource management, and leadership" (p. 106). From their work, the debriefing session is the opportunity for the faculty to develop and support the ability of the student to "think like a nurse." It is during these sessions where the positive aspects of the interactions must be recognized and developed.

Thomas Dreifuerst (2009) completed extensive work examining the debriefing process. The evidence relates the debriefing session as "the process whereby faculty and students reexamine the clinical encounter, fosters the development of clinical reasoning and judgment skills through reflective learning processes" (p. 109). It is during this session that the faculty embraces the opportunity to support and develop the student cohort in a positive manner. Thomas Dreifuerst (2009) established five objectives for the debriefing process:

1. identification of the different perceptions and attitudes that have occurred;
2. linking the exercise to specific theory or content and skill-building techniques;
3. development of a common set of experiences for further thought;
4. opportunity to receive feedback on the nature of one's involvement, behavior, and decision making; and
5. reestablishment of the desired classroom climate, such as regaining trust, comfort, and purposefulness. (p. 110)

Faculty members need to carefully consider these five aspects as they strive to come to grips with the idea of debriefing. The debriefing session should be provided to facilitate the students' best learning opportunity. As a result, faculty members need to understand how important this part of the learning process is. Thomas Dreifuerst (2009) found that the attributes of reflection, emotion, reception, integration, and assimilation were the defining attributes of simulation debriefing. When these five attributes are carefully considered by the faculty, the debriefing sessions can be an effective teaching/learning situation. Reflection is viewed as an occasion to retrace the experience. During this aspect, the group takes times to come to agreement about what actually happened during the experience. It is a listing of the different processes that occurred—a timeline of the case. Next, the connected emotions and emotional release are important to verbalize. As students engage in the scenario, emotions become an integral part of the process. Emotions related to past experiences may be encountered by some of the students. Emotions related to the process may also be encountered. As each member assumes a role within the scenario, emotions can result. The debriefing process should address these emotions and allow the student group to work through them. Reception, or openness to feedback, is a crucial aspect of learning. Simulation experiences embrace cognitive, affective, and psychomotor skills. All of the participants should be expected to provide feedback on those skills from their viewpoints. During the debriefing session, the views of each person should be acknowledged and considered to provide an inclusive view of the experience. According to Thomas Dreifuerst (2009), "integration of the simulation experience and the facilitated reflection into a conceptual framework is one of the most challenging and least common attributes of debriefing" (p. 111). This process of bringing all of the parts together to enable the student to understand the complexity of healthcare delivery is of paramount importance. According to Thomas Dreifuerst (2009), the components of the simulation experience "link the experience to the curriculum, guide the facilitation of the debriefing discussion, and provide structure for evaluating the experience" (p. 113). Within the conducting of the debriefing, each student and each learning objective along with the multicomplexity of the clinical scenario should be carefully and completely discussed to allow for the development of a firm foundation of nursing knowledge. The debriefing is viewed as a fundamental and essential component within the clinical simulation experience. It closes the loop on the learning process and allows the students to connect the different pieces, both negative and positive, into a learning opportunity.

The final piece of evidence presented here is focused on the faculty member and was presented by Dillard, Sideras, Ryan, Hodson-Carlton, Lasater, and Siktberg (2009). An urgent need was identified that faculty members require faculty development opportunities related to the development of the new pedagogical skills necessary for the management of the complex pieces of technology involved in HFS. To expect faculty members to already have the skills needed to effectively organize, manage, and facilitate clinical simulation experiences is inappropriate. The skill set needed to be applicable to this type of clinical experience requires the faculty members to update their knowledge and thought processes. Because the faculty/student ratios utilized within the clinical settings do not consistently allow faculty members time to adequately observe the students as they attempt to make clinical judgments, clinical simulation experiences are viewed as a means to overcome this deficiency by allowing sufficient time to observe each student's clinical judgment process. Dillard et al. (2009) found that "HFS allows for a more comprehensive evaluation of the development of students' clinical judgment as well as recognition of gaps in their understanding of clinical practice" (p. 100). HFS and other clinical simulations focus on the outcomes. As a result, faculty members have to convert their thought processes for clinical experiences to the idea of outcomes. This conversion of thought compels the faculty members to re-conceptualize the pedagogy of teaching as it relates to simulation implementation and linking learning from simulation opportunities to clinical practice. According to Dillard et al. (2009), "no standardized curriculum has yet been developed for simulation use" (p. 103). In addition to the lack of a standardized curriculum, a consistent technique for appraising student learning in simulation is also nonexistent. Thus, the evaluation aspect of simulation experiences needs to be carefully and thoughtfully discussed and envisioned.

Evidence is present for the incorporation of clinical simulation as a means for addressing the clinical knowledge needed to conduct health care. Ongoing research is also being done to further clarify the roles and expectations needed to effectively conduct the acquisition of nursing knowledge related to the clinical setting.

Types of Clinical Strategies

Many nurses and other healthcare providers have not actively incorporated research findings into clinical practice settings. In fact, until recently, many nurses were aware of research but had not shifted the research into their practices. Melnyk and Fineout-Overhold (2005) report that research utilization is the use of research knowledge from a single study for clinical practice. Evidence-based practice (EBP) involves: (a) best evidence from a thorough search and critical appraisal of all studies, (b) context, (c) healthcare resources, (d) patient status and individual circumstances, and (e) what the client values and prefers for his or her care.

Educators, **preceptors**, and **coaches** can adapt the following steps to incorporate EBP into their specific clinical settings: (1) Formulate a clinical question to be researched; (2) systematically search for relevant research/evidence that either supports or disputes the specific clinical practice; (3) evaluate the relevance, quality, and application to the practice setting; (4) determine the evidence-based decision through consideration of the research/evidence compiled; (5) couple the research/evidence with the practitioners' clinical experiences and expertise and resources; (6) apply to the patient's clinical status and preferences that support the specific action; (7) implement the change within the practice setting; and (8) evaluate the outcome of the clinical change through systematic EBP (DiCenso, Cullum, Ciliska, & Guyatt, 2004). Clinical reasoning strategies to provide guidance for specific student clinical questions should be prioritized through the evidence-based process for both the hospital bedside and community clinical office settings. When students recognize the process of incorporating EBP within their settings, optimal provision of healthcare services will occur.

Traditionally, clinical faculties have utilized care plans, care maps, and clinical logs to evaluate students' growth. Today, preceptors or coaches are used to facilitate: (a) a "hands-on" approach that includes teaching microskills, (b) observation of their skill sets by being observed or shadowed by their students, (c) provision of mini-lectures on skills and clinical processes, (d) mentoring of students through clinical projects, and, finally, (e) "learning" vicariously through their students' research on projects and papers. Through utilization of a mixture of methods, education will likely be more enjoyable and effective to facilitate maximum clinical growth for the student (DiCenso et al., 2004). Hands-on approaches will provide solid interventional strategies through clinical reasoning that is based on current evidence and guidelines.

Conducting clinical experiences at the undergraduate setting requires more face-to-face time with clinical faculty members. Since these students are novice healthcare providers, time and energy must be given to ensuring that they develop the foundation needed to provide safe and practical health care. The faculty member's energy is directed toward providing appropriate and adequate clinical opportunities for each student to develop clinical expertise while ensuring that critical thinking opportunities are presented. Care must be taken in relation to the clinical experience as to which skills, tasks, and/or opportunities must be provided to ensure that the students are competent following the conclusion of the clinical process. Each and every student will not be afforded the same exact opportunities, so the drive is to determine which aspects must be provided at which level and setting. Another aspect of the clinical experience relates to the thought process being developed. Determinations of the types of assignments are needed to reflect and ensure that the students develop the appropriate clinical decision-making skills. Most daily teaching should include the combination of: (1) precepting using "microskills," (2) being observed or shadowed by the student, (3) observation of the student, (4) giving "mini-lectures," (5) mentoring student projects with application of evidence-based clinical practice guidelines and research studies, and (6) learning together with the student as both the preceptor/coach and student search the Internet, clinical resources, or texts for answers to clinical questions. These clinical decision-making skills can then be incorporated into other clinical settings.

Teaching while practicing on busy days can be challenging, but the reality is that every day is a busy day. Effective preceptors and coaches prepare ahead for the day and include specific strategies for success. Prior to the beginning of the rotation, it is helpful to actually meet the student and determine his or her objectives, goals, learning style, and past experiences prior to this experience. All members of the practice setting need to meet the student and discuss the clinical strategy. To have optimal success for the student and the agency, scheduling of patients, experiences desired, examination room availability, a documentation area, and planning for the student to have access to patient records is necessary (DiCenso et al., 2004). To facilitate immersion of students in the clinical setting, an identified workspace should be arranged for the students' use of their texts, references, and computers, thus facilitating the learning experience for the student. As complexities increase with new health issues, students can utilize a 5-minute online consult that brings evidence into their specific clinical practice experiences. Golway (2008) reports that the focus of the 2008 Accreditation Symposium for American Nursing Credentialing Center was to question if evidenced based approaches were guiding teaching in nursing. Their recommendation was to adopt the evidence-based approach to teach by these four steps: (1) question your own teaching practices, (2) search for evidence to answer questions, (3) decide if findings are applicable to your own teaching situation, and (4) use evidence to guide teaching. Ideally, the student workspace would emulate the workspace provided for the preceptor/coach to facilitate immersion of the students to maximize clinical learning, and application of both teaching and student EBP activities.

Clinical expertise, teaching style, and philosophy of patient care can be provided by the preceptor. This should provide a focus of the actual services provided within the specific clinical setting. Coverage of the agency's mission, patients served, standards, and guidelines that the site has incorporated will facilitate clinical practitioner roles as well as expected student behaviors. Prior to clinical activities, students should be introduced to the organization of the clinic, including the reception area, patient/staff restrooms, laboratory, clinical rooms, procedure rooms, and staff offices. This introduction will facilitate student familiarity prior to the first day of the clinical experiences, resulting in reduction in stress for both clinical staff and the student.

Daily clinical schedules should be provided for the student when arriving for clinical experiences, and a short post-clinical reflection at the end of the experience will identify specific professional growth and challenges on a daily basis. Consideration should be given to request the students to examine one to two clinical case studies based on the specific challenges they have experienced. When students report their research findings, utilization of evidence-based research studies and clinical guidelines should be stressed. As student nurses, preceptors, coaches, and other healthcare providers adapt evidence-based clinical guidelines and research into daily clinical practice settings, solid patient care will be provided to their patients.

Student Evaluation

Teachers and preceptors/coaches share the responsibility of monitoring the progress of students by analyzing specific clinical activities, types of patients seen, complexity of health issues, procedural activities, and application of case studies for provision of solid, evidence-based practice. Evaluation can be done through a variety of venues, including: (1) clinical schedules and patients seen; (2) individualized contracts with preceptors/coaches based on their area of expertise; (3) development of specific clinical goals that are measurable and appropriate for the courses being taken; (4) review of written goals by the student, preceptor/coach, and clinical faculty to evaluate the students' growth; (5) clinical performance scores through measurement tools utilized by preceptors/coaches and clinical faculty; (6) successful site visits where students, preceptors/coaches, and faculty meet face-to-face to observe and discuss progress of students; (7) successful clinical performance by students with faculty members; and (8) final course evaluations by preceptors/coaches and clinical faculty to determine specific competencies obtained during the course of the semester. Opportunities should be provided to students to evaluate the clinical site where they have worked, their preceptors/coaches, the effectiveness of their clinical experience, and the support from their clinical faculty. Gaberson and Oermann (1999) support the triad of clinical experiences the student, preceptor/coach, and clinical faculty have participated in and evaluation to determine clinical outcomes.

Evaluation of student complexities includes issues such as the variety of preceptor/coach working hours, specific clinical locations, preceptor/coaching expertise, student work schedules, and family responsibilities. Evaluation of clinical experiences can no longer always be done face-to-face in the classroom setting. Ongoing evaluation must be done through a mixture of experiences, such as telephone contact, emails, online chat rooms, and face-to-face contact in specific clinical settings. Contact between the preceptor/coach and the clinical faculty is also imperative to offset challenges the students may have within their clinical setting. When preceptors/coaches provide feedback concerning learner performance, the clinical faculty can offer guidance and recommendations based on their expertise. Challenges can be daunting, time consuming, and expensive for course faculty, preceptors/coaches, colleges, and universities as they guide their students through their clinical activities.

In hospital settings, clinical evaluations should focus on clinical standards such as professional behavior, professional integrity, patient-centered care, interdisciplinary care, quality improvement, informatics, and patient safety, with EBP as the foundation for clinical judgment utilized to guide specific clinical decisions. Coaches and faculty members should provide evaluation based on the ability to communicate with patients and families, cultural and health beliefs of patients and families, and specific contributions to coordination of patient care that utilize the nursing process framework within the current evidence guidelines. Finally, attention should encompass patient safety in terms of safe and effective patient-centered care, provision of care in a timely manner, and identification and reduction of risks to patients.

Summary Thoughts

Clinical experiences must always be a component of nursing education. The question becomes one of how such experiences can be effectively and efficiently managed. Though actual care of clients is paramount and should never be completely removed from the educational process, clinical simulation is one way to gain the best out of the process during times when availability is compromised. According to Taglareni (2009), "new technologies and changing patient demographics require our graduates to work quickly, efficiently, and safely, and to think and act in ways that reach far beyond current practice realities" (p. 69). Simulation embraces the undertaking of transforming faculty members' beliefs about how students discover and deliberate while becoming an indispensable teaching/assessment/evaluation strategy in the education of nurses.

With appropriate clinical strategies and evaluation methodologies, most nurses with extensive clinical experiences can and do serve as excellent preceptors/coaches. Utilization of evidence-based educational strategies includes: (a) continuous pre-planning, (b) provision of student time with patients, (c) facilitation of challenging patient case presentations, and (d) post-clinical discussion times. Students, preceptors, and coaches will readily be able to easily recognize each student's clinical growth and challenges (Burns, Beauchesne, Ryan-Krause, & Sawin, 2008). Preceptors and coaches are and will continue to be the front line for training the future generations of nurses through access to clinical sites, patients, expert mentoring, and sharing of clinical experiences to facilitate students' clinical growth.

Summary Points

1. An ideal clinical setting is one that presents encounters that are applicable, pertinent, and timely for the content being presented within the courses and that sanction persistent reinforcement and practice for the skills already acquired.

2. Evidence-based teaching must strive to locate the best evidence instead of depending on the patterns used over the decades.

3. The ultimate criterion for the learning process within the clinical setting is the acquisition of skills in a timely manner while supporting and confirming skills already learned.

4. With the complexities of the patient population, simulation activities allow students to acquire knowledge with situations prior to being placed in that setting.

5. By having the opportunities to work through problems with the use of a device, students and faculty members can provide educational materials, evaluate the different options, and incorporate research/evidence while in a safe, nonthreatening environment.

6. As individuals take an active part in the learning process, genuine, meaningful and long-lasting learning occurs.

7. As a person develops self-efficacy and self-confidence, he or she becomes adept at confronting challenges successfully, seeking learning opportunities, developing commitment to the learning process, and recovering promptly from obstacles and disappointments.

8. Because the simulation situation is controlled by the faculty members involved, the depth of the clinical situation with the incorporation of key knowledge points can be managed and addressed during the simulation experience prior to the student confronting the aspects within a real-world setting.

9. Static manikins restrict the learning to one narrow task practice.

10. Moderate-fidelity simulators are those models that are two-dimensional in their focus on the experiences being learned.

11. With high-fidelity simulators, case presentations can be complicated and in-depth.

12. High-fidelity simulations incorporate the resolution of problems, advance teamwork, facilitate a better understanding of complex disease problems, and support decision making and critical thinking.

13. Clinical simulation provides opportunities for students to apply their didactic knowledge and problem-solving skills, critical thinking abilities, and time management skills.

14. Simulation allows the faculty member to adjust variations based upon the current healthcare arena.

15. Simulation has been found to endorse the skills of communication, teamwork, delegation, priority setting, and leadership.

16. Debriefing sessions are a key component within the simulation process. During these sessions, faculty members must help the students to examine the case and analyze the clinical reasoning and judgment skills used during the process.

17. During debriefing, each student and each learning objective along with the multiplicity of the clinical scenario should be carefully and completely discussed to allow for the development of a firm foundation of nursing knowledge.

18. Faculty members require faculty development opportunities related to the development of new pedagogical skills needed to manage the complex pieces of technology involved in HFS.

19. Principles of clinical teaching include: (1) learning is evolutionary and occurs from both a student and preceptor/coach focus; (2) participation, repetition, and reinforcement facilitate student learning; (3) various aspects of clinical experiences increase role satisfaction for students and preceptors/coaches; and (4) use of clinical guidelines and evidence-based studies enhances clinical expertise and provision of care.

20. Both student and preceptor/coach satisfaction will increase through pre-planning and ongoing clinical experience planning to facilitate maximum student experiences.

21. Utilization of evidence-based clinical teaching will provide mentorship to students and facilitate their use of current clinical guidelines and evidence-based applications for provision of patient care.

Tips for Nurse Educators to Use

1. Clinical experiences must be carefully planned and organized to gain the utmost positive outcome for the students. The agency, unit, personnel, and objectives for the clinical experience must be thoughtfully considered.

2. Clinical simulation is one strategy for addressing clinical skills and knowledge.

3. High-fidelity simulation requires focused preparation time from both the faculty member and the students.

4. Student planning time should be included in the time allotted for simulation experiences to gain the maximum results from the opportunity.

5. The debriefing session for each clinical encounter should be carefully planned and orchestrated for the optimum outcome. Within each session, the clinical objectives should be addressed so that students understand where within the course materials the experience is directed.

6. Provision of student work areas within the clinical setting is integral to having texts, computers, and learning materials readily available for student use.

7. Access to resources will provide learning environments that link didactic and clinical strategies for optimal patient care.
8. Teaching strategy options should include utilization of clinical case presentations based on the direct clinical experiences of the day. Both open-ended and direct questioning can facilitate the critical thinking processes.
9. Student assignments between clinical experiences should facilitate EBP through use of the most recent clinical guidelines and research studies that support the care the students provide to their patients.

References

Adams, M. H., & Valiga, T. M. (2009). Achieving excellence in nursing education. New York, NY: National League for Nursing.

Bambino, D., Washington, J., & Perkins, R. (2009). Outcomes of clinical simulation for novice nursing students: Communication, confidence, clinical judgment. *Nursing Education Perspectives* 30(2), 79–82.

Benner, P. (1984). *From novice to expert.* Menlo Park, CA: Addison-Wesley.

Burns, C., Beauchesne, M., Ryan-Krause, P., & Sawin, K. (2008). Mastering the preceptor role: Challenges of clinical teaching. *Journal of Pediatric Health Care,* 20(3), 172–183.

Cato, M. L., Lasater, K., & Peeples, A. I. (2009). Nursing students' self-assessment of their simulation experiences. *Nursing Education Perspectives,* 30(2), 105–108.

DiCenso, A., Cullum, N., Ciliska, D., & Guyatt, G. (2004). *Evidence-based nursing: A guide to clinical practice.* Philadelphia, PA: Elsevier.

Dillard, N., Sideras, S., Ryan, M., Hodson-Carlton, K., Lasater, K., & Siktberg, L. (2009). A collaborative project to apply and evaluate the clinical judgment model through simulation. *Nursing Education Perspectives,* 30(2), 99–104.

Dillon, P. M., Noble, K. A., & Kaplan, L. (2009). Simulation as a means to foster collaborative interdisciplinary education. *Nursing Education Perspectives,* 30(2), 87–90.

Elfrink, V. L., Nininger, J., Rohig, L., & Lee, J. (2009). The case for group planning in human patient simulation. *Nursing Education Perspectives,* 30(2), 83–86.

Gaberson, K. B., & Oermann, M. H. (1999). *Clinical teaching strategies in nursing.* New York, NY: Springer.

Golway, J. (2008). Conference report-2008 accreditation symposium: Is an evidence-based approach guiding teaching in nursing? *American Nurses Credentialing Center.* Retrieved February 26, 2010, from www.medscape.com

Hoadley, T. A. (2009). Learning advanced cardiac life support: A comparison study of the effects of low- and high-fidelity simulation. *Nursing Education Perspectives,* 30(2), 91–95.

Jeffries, P. R. (2008). The three E's: Effective, engaging, and evidence-based teaching using simulation. PNEG 2008 Conference.

Jeffries, P. R. (2009). Dreams for the future for clinical simulation. *Nursing Education Perspectives,* 30(2), 71.

Letvak, S. (2008). Developing new clinical experiences for students. In B. K. Penn (Ed.), *Mastering the teaching role: A guide for nurse educators* (pp. 191–199). Philadelphia, PA: F.A. Davis.

Melynk, B. M., & Fineout-Overholt, E. (2005). *Evidence-based practice in nursing and healthcare* (pp. 186-216). Philadelphia, PA.: Lippincott Williams & Wilkins.

Misener, T (2008). Strategic relationships with clinical agencies. In B. K. Penn (Ed.), *Mastering the teaching role: A guide for nurse educators* (pp. 179–190). Philadelphia, PA: F.A. Davis.

Neill, J. (2005). What is experiential learning? Retrieved December 30, 2009, from www.wilderdom.com/experiential/ExperientialLearningWhatIs.html

Simulation Innovation and Resource Center. (n.d.). SIRC glossary—Static manikin. Retrieved December 30, 2009, from http://sirc.nln.org/mod/glossary/view.php

Smith, M. M. (2009). Creative clinical solutions: Aligning simulation with authentic clinical experiences. *Nursing Education Perspectives, 30*(2), 126–127.

Smith, S. J., & Roehrs, C. J. (2009). High-fidelity simulation: Factors correlated with nursing student satisfaction and self-confidence. *Nursing Education Perspectives, 30*(2), 74–78.

Spunt, D., & Covington, B. G. (2008). Utilizing clinical simulation. In B. K. Penn (Ed.), *Mastering the teaching role: A guide for nurse educators* (pp. 233–251). Philadelphia, PA: F.A. Davis.

Tagliareni, M. E. (2009). Beyond the realities of current practice: Preparing students to provide safe and effective care. *Nursing Education Perspectives, 30*(2), 69.

ThinkQuest Team. (n.d.). 5. Cognitive processes. Retrieved December 30, 2009, from http://library.thinkquest.org/26618/en-5.5.3=cognitive%20learning.htm

Thomas Dreifuerst, K. (2009). The essentials of debriefing in simulation learning: A concept analysis. *Nursing Education Perspectives, 30*(2), 109–114.

Van Wagner, K. (n.d.). What is self-efficacy? Retrieved December 30, 2009, from http://psychology.about.com/od/theoriesofpersonality/a/self-efficacy.htm

Web Links

The Simulation Innovation and Resource Center (SIRC) of the NLN and Laerdal Medical site is available at http://sirc.nln.org.

View the home page of the National Guideline Clearinghouse at www.guideline.gov.

View the Evidence-Based Teaching site (under development) at http://evidencebasedteaching.com.

Multiple Choice Questions

1. The primary reason for utilizing clinical experiences with students is the

    A. timely acquisition of skills and confirmation of previously learned skills.

    B. management of clinical skills for management of the education experience.

    C. timely acquisition of skills without the need for further follow-up.

    D. supporting and confirming of previously learned skills only.

Rationale:

No matter the location of the clinical experience provided or what resources are used, the ultimate criterion for the learning process is the acquisition of skills in a timely manner while also supporting and confirming skills already learned.

2. Experiential learning is understood to mean learning that

    A. is completed within a specific site or location.

    B. is completed by a person or through a program/activity structured by others.

    C. is completed by a person without structure from another person.

    D. results from a program that is directed by the individual.

Rationale:

Experiential learning implies that the learning is done by a person or through a program/activity structured by others (Neill, 2005). Within this form of learning the emphasis is placed on active participation by all members involved (Thomas Dreifuerst, 2009). As individuals take an active part in the learning process, genuine, meaningful, and long-lasting learning occurs.

3. The simulators referred to as human patient simulators are

    A. low-fidelity simulators, moderate-fidelity simulators, and high-fidelity simulators.

    B. moderate-fidelity simulators and high-fidelity simulators.

    C. static manikins, moderate-fidelity simulators, and high-fidelity simulators.

    D. low-fidelity simulators and high-fidelity simulators.

Rationale:

According to Adams and Valiga (2009), "high fidelity and medium [moderate] fidelity simulators are life-like mannequins, referred to as human patient simulators that are programmed to mimic the responses of a human being" (p. 100). Moderate-fidelity simulators are those models that are two-dimensional in their focus on the experience being learned. This level of simulator encourages problem solving within the management of the manikin case study. Spunt and Covington (2009) note that "high-fidelity simulation offers the most realistic clinical experience possible, short of caring for a real patient, and may involve advanced equipment that interacts with the learner" (p. 234). With the high-fidelity simulators, the case presentations can be complicated and in-depth.

4. Simulation and simulated case scenarios are effective means for appraising and examining

   A.   didactic skills, critical thinking, clinical judgment, time management, delegation, communication skills, and leadership only.
   B.   didactic skills, critical thinking, clinical judgment, and leadership only.
   C.   clinical skills, critical thinking, clinical judgment, time management, delegation, communication skills, and leadership.
   D.   clinical skills only.

Rationale:

Adams and Valiga (2009) stated that simulation and simulated case scenarios are an effective means for appraising and examining clinical skills, critical thinking, and clinical judgments within the context of re-creating healthcare needs from a client's viewpoint. Cato et al. (2009) state that the "debriefing that follows each scenario focuses on the team's care of the patient, including safe practice, priority setting, continuous assessment, communication, resource management, and leadership" (p. 106). From the work done by this team of researchers, simulation was found to endorse the skills of communication, teamwork, delegation, priority setting, and leadership.

5. Research has shown simulations to be effective at

   A.   incorporating the management of problems, discouraging teamwork, facilitating an improved understanding of complex disease problems, and augmenting decision making and critical thinking.
   B.   incorporating the solving of problems, encouraging teamwork, restricting understanding of complex disease problems, and augmenting decision making and critical thinking.
   C.   incorporating the management of problems, encouraging teamwork, facilitating an improved understanding of only simple disease problems, and augmenting decision making and critical thinking.
   incorporating the solving of problems, encouraging teamwork, facilitating an improved understanding of complex disease problems, and augmenting decision making and critical thinking.

Rationale:

Smith (2009) relates that HFS activities within skills labs are predominantly used to ensure the learning of skills and tasks. Smith goes on to say that the use of HFS within a simulated clinical setting incorporates the solving of problems, encourages teamwork, facilitates a better understanding of complex disease problems, and augments decision making and critical thinking.

6. One advantage identified with the use of simulations is that it
   A. restricts faculty members from making variations in the case study based upon current healthcare issues and practices.
   B. allows faculty members to make variations in the case study based upon current healthcare issues and practices.
   C. allows students to make variations in the case study based upon current healthcare issues and practices.
   D. allows faculty members to hold constant any variations in the case study for consistency.

Rationale:

Simulations allow faculty members to make variations to case studies based upon the current healthcare arena. As new and innovative changes are encountered in the workplace, changes can be made to the scenarios to address them. Also, as political changes occur, such as in the national health care policy, these aspects can be incorporated into the scenario to allow for currency of the educational process.

7. As an experiential learning technique and strategy, simulation promotes the cohort to
   A. associate applicable concepts, employ suitable theories in clinical practice, and determine satisfactory clinical decisions.
   B. associate applicable concepts, contrast suitable theories to clinical practice, and restrict the formation of clinical decisions.
   C. associate of concepts, employ all theories to clinical practice, and determine some clinical decisions.
   D. associate applicable strategies, employ all theories to clinical practice, and determine satisfactory clinical decisions.

Rationale:

As an experiential learning technique and strategy, simulation promotes the cohort to associate the applicable concepts, employ suitable theories in clinical practice, and determine satisfactory clinical decisions. From the work done by this team of researchers, simulation was found to enhance the skills of communication, teamwork, delegation, priority setting, and leadership.

8. Debriefing sessions used following a simulation period serve as an opportunity for
   A. faculty members to develop and support students to "think like a student."

  B. students to develop and support each other to "think like a nurse."
  C. **faculty members to develop and support students to "think like a nurse."**
  D. faculty members to develop and support students to "think like a physician."

Rationale:

Cato et al. (2009) state that the "debriefing that follows each scenario focuses on the team's care of the patient, including safe practice, priority setting, continuous assessment, communication, resource management, and leadership" (p. 106). From their work, the debriefing session is characterized as the opportunity for the faculty to develop and support the ability of the student to "think like a nurse." It is during these sessions where the positive aspects of the interactions must be recognized and developed.

9. The debriefing session should address:

  A. **course objectives, the timeline, resulting emotions, integration of key concepts, and feedback.**
  B. course objectives only.
  C. problems encountered during the session and what the students should have done.
  D. mistakes identified and areas not addressed.

Rationale:

Thomas Dreifuerst (2009) found that the attributes of reflection, emotion, reception, integration, and assimilation were the defining characteristics of simulation debriefing. During the debriefing session, the views of each person should be acknowledged and considered to provide an inclusive view of the experience. This process brings all of the parts together to aid the student to understand that the complexity of healthcare delivery is of paramount importance. According to Thomas Dreifuerst (2009), the attributes "link the experience to the curriculum, guide the facilitation of the debriefing discussion, and provide structure for evaluating the experience" (p. 113). Within the conduction of the debriefing, each student and each learning objective along with the multiplicity of the clinical scenario should be carefully and completely discussed to allow for the development of a firm foundation of nursing knowledge. The debriefing is viewed as a fundamental and essential component within the clinical simulation experience. It closes the loop in the learning process and allows the students to connect the different pieces, both negative and positive, into a learning opportunity.

10. As faculty members move toward the use of clinical simulations, the thought and evaluation processes need to move toward

    A. faculty development.
    B. outcomes.
    C. pre-planning.
    D. shortcomings in the curriculum.

Rationale:

High-fidelity simulations and other clinical simulations focus on the outcomes. As a result, faculty members have to convert their thought processes for clinical experiences to the idea of outcomes.

11. One strategy preceptors can use to facilitate maximum student learning while maintaining patient loads in clinical settings is

    A. reducing the client flow for the student's clinical day.
    B. having the student "jump in," with little discussion of student expectations.
    C. utilizing pre-planning and continuous planning prior to student arrival,
    D. d. having the student follow the preceptor throughout the entire day.

Rationale:

Burns et al. (2008) indicate that to be successful on a busy day, it is essential to pre-plan the day. This includes having the student arrive prior to the day of the clinical experience to meet the staff, review student objectives, learn the charting for the clinical setting, and learn the layout of the setting. This will facilitate increased comfort for the preceptor, staff, and student.

12. The recommended evidence-based approach to teaching includes all of the following, *except*

    A. use evidence to guide clinical-based teaching.
    B. question your own clinical practice.
    C. search for evidence to answer specific clinical questions.
    D. save research activities until after clinical experiences.

Rationale:

Golway (2008) reports that the focus of the 2008 Accreditation Symposium for American Nursing Credentialing Center was to question if evidenced based approaches were guiding teaching in nursing. Their recommendation was to adopt the evidence-based approach to teach by these four steps: (1) question your own teaching practices, (2) search for evidence to answer questions, (3) decide if findings are applicable to your own teaching situation, and (4) use evidence to guide teaching.

13. To evaluate the teaching day, the preceptor/coach and student should

    A.   provide a written list of concerns prior to leaving for the day.

    B.   have the clinic staff evaluate the effectiveness of the student.

    C.   think briefly about who was seen, what was accomplished, and how the student felt.

    D.   ask the patients how the patient encounter went.

Rationale:

Evaluation of the day should occur routinely and focus on who was seen, what was done, how the student felt about the experience, where the student wants to go next in terms of experiences, and why things worked/didn't work. Through critical reflection on the day's experiences, both the preceptor/coach and student can determine the next clinical day's activities.

14. Teaching that incorporates utilization of microskills, shadowing, observation, mini-lectures, mentoring, and use of Internet, clinical resources, and texts is an effective strategy in

    A.   research arenas.

    B.   evidence-based practice.

    C.   classroom activities.

    D.   educational projects.

Rationale:

Most daily teaching will include the combination of: (1) precepting using "microskills," (2) being observed or shadowed by the student, (3) observation of the student, (4) giving "mini-lectures," (5) mentoring student projects with application of evidence-based clinical practice guidelines and research studies, and (6) learning together with the student as both the preceptor/coach and student search the Internet, clinical resources, or texts for answers to clinical questions.

15. The best use of evidence to guide complex clinical teaching includes

    A.   using clinical experiences of the day to facilitate learning.

    B.   lecturing the student about difficult clinical experiences encountered.

    C.   having both the preceptor and student research recommended treatments.

    D.   asking the student to verify specific clinical experiences obtained.

Rationale:

To support a higher level of questioning and stimulate learning, analyze and utilize critical thinking through research that both the preceptor and student work on together. This experience will bring to the table clinical expertise and student questioning of the validity of treatments used.

Discussion Questions

1. Is a solid, evidence-based approach currently being utilized to guide teaching in nursing?

Considerations:

- Are traditional approaches in clinical teaching effective?
- Do we question our own teaching practices?
- Is the teaching technique for searching the evidence appropriate or practical?
- Are evidence-based guidelines applicable to your own teaching situation?
- How can you use evidence to guide your teaching?
- From Golway (2008).

2. What are the role expectations for the student, faculty, and preceptor?

Considerations:

- Student expectations: student role pressures, including connections between didactic and clinical work
- Faculty expectations: identification and securing of appropriate sites/ preceptors in a time of preceptor shortage; support of preceptor to facilitate student learning experiences
- Preceptor expectations: provision of course objectives for student clinical experiences; how preceptors can provide informal, collaborative, respectful, and challenging learning environments
- From Burns et al. (2008).

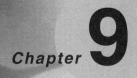

Chapter **9**

Program Evaluation

Patricia Allen and Carol Boswell

Chapter Objectives

At the conclusion of this chapter, the learner will be able to:

1. Differentiate the strengths and limitations of different evaluation models.
2. Describe different aspects inherent in the accreditation process.
3. Summarize key characteristics found within a program evaluation process.
4. Discuss crucial facets necessary for effective course evaluation.
5. Recognize significant aspects within the evaluation of faculty members.

Key Terms

- ➤ Evaluation models
- ➤ Formative evaluation
- ➤ Gap analysis
- ➤ Professional or national accreditation

- ➤ Program evaluation
- ➤ Regional accreditation
- ➤ Regulatory agency
- ➤ Summative evaluation

Introduction

Evidence-based practice (EBP) is the underpinning for excellence in nursing practice resulting in quality nurses and improved patient outcomes. According to Newhouse and Johnson (2009), "the evaluation of the work context for readiness for EBP is the first step to laying the groundwork to successfully build the structures and processes needed to support decision making by nurses in the organization" (p. 409). In nursing education, the drive toward quality and excellence must be founded on evidence-based teaching (EBT) aspects in the same manner as nursing practice is based upon EBP. The transition to using evidence to propel and empower nursing education is viewed as a natural progression toward excellence. By considering the evidence for each aspect within the educational process, the educational community will advance the profession to an exceptional and enhanced delivery of the key components within the process. Because evaluation is a crucial facet within this process, it must be carefully and thoroughly discussed and incorporated into the process of EBT.

Evaluation has an impact on every aspect within the educational process. According to Oermann, Saewert, Charasika, and Yarbrough (2009b), "evaluation is both the process of systematic collection and interpretation of data gathered from multiple sources about clinical competence and the product or outcome of that process – the decision about whether the student has passed the course" (p. 353). This process of systematically collecting, analyzing, and interpreting data to aid in the determination of quality educational outcomes is crucial for the establishment and management of effective nursing programs. Every aspect within the educational program is open to evaluation.

According to Lowenstein and Bradshaw (2004), "faculty members are also involved in evaluation of teaching, evaluation of their peers, and evaluation of the program" (p. 349). Accreditation agencies mandate that each facet of a program be carefully, methodically, and logically appraised to reflect the quality of the programmatic goals and outcomes designated within the program. Within this process, administration, faculty, curriculum, and students are all assessed to determine their unique parts within the advancement of a quality program of study resulting in highly qualified students ready to assume the role of competent entry-level registered nurse. This chapter will provide insight into the multiplicity of the evaluation process as it relates to the educational setting.

Evaluation Models

Evaluation models have been in use by educators for the past 150 years. The first noted evaluation model began when a principal in Boston compared student test scores to gain insight into the test questions and how effective the test was in capturing student knowledge. Next, the U.S. military began to have uniformity policies for all arms manufacturing, and arms were evaluated for adherence to uniformity measures (Stufflebeam, Madaus, & Kellaghan, 2000). It is essential that faculty are able to document change through both formal and informal methods. Crucial to documentation is designing and using evaluative tools and methods to enhance feedback. Though this process of formal and informal methods of evaluation can be traced back 150 years, the push for development of knowledge in the field of evaluation began with earnest in the Johnson administration with the "Great Society," where government pushed for accountability in areas of federal laws for equitable services for the disabled and minorities. Program evaluation continued to grow in the 1970s to hold social organizations accountable for resource use. In the 1980s, evaluation focused on excellence as a method of increasing international competiveness. Finally, in the 1990s, industry engaged in evaluation as a means of improving quality.

Evaluation provides the evidence needed for delivering effective teaching methodologies, curricula, and program development. Strong methods of evaluation are needed to yield accurate evidence for creating, critiquing, and revising current programs. Evaluation is the anchor of the growing "science of quality" that monitors and assures the quality of selected methods, curricula, and programs. Evaluation models are used to help define the characteristic or features of an evaluation, what concepts to study, and the processes or methods needed to extract critical data, evidence, and outcomes. A brief review of widely used evaluation models was obtained from Virginia Tech (2009) and includes the following:

- **Connoisseurship Evaluation (Eisner, 1976)**: involves an expert in the discipline of study estimating the value of a new innovation. Obvious biases and threats to validity can be seen in this approach to evaluation.
- **Goals-Oriented/Objectives-Based (Tyler, 1949)**: describes whether or not students have met their goals and objectives,

with the results suggesting how to handle a new instructional strategy (i.e., revise, adopt, reject). One shortfall may be that the evaluator may overlook unexpected outcomes or benefits of instruction beyond original goals and objectives. This is one of earliest models of evaluation used in nursing education. Tyler's model was widely used in nursing education in the 1960s and 1970s.

▪ **Goals-Free Evaluation (Scriven, 1972)**: supplements inherent weaknesses in a goals-oriented approach by providing an unbiased tracking of ongoing events. This model uses a checklist beginning with a needs assessment, then noting comparative value, and then assessment of overall value. Evaluators are encouraged to use this checklist with three columns comparing need, comparative value, and overall value.

▪ **Judicial/Adversary Evaluation (Worthen, Sanders, & Fitzpatrick, 1997)**: focuses on comparing or describing all sides of a program, both strengths and weaknesses. It is compared to the defense and prosecution of a courtroom because the potential for evaluation bias by a single evaluator cannot be ruled out. To deter bias, each "side" has an evaluator to make its case.

▪ **Kirkpatrick's Four-Level Model (Kirkpatrick, 1998)**: describes student reactions to and learning from an event, program, or innovation, as well as perceived or observed changes in performance. The four levels are reaction, learning, behavior, and results. This model is used in training programs.

▪ **Situated Evaluation (Bruce & Rubin, 1993)**: is a contextual model for evaluation. Here the characteristics of varying contexts that cause programs to fail or succeed are reviewed. Proponents of situated evaluation argue that educational events, programs, and training are situated within their context of use; therefore, context cannot be overlooked.

▪ **Stufflebeam's CIPP Model (2002)**: describes the context in which an innovation occurs, the inputs of the innovation, the formative processes occurring, and the summative products or outcomes. The CIPP model flows from a checklist format where the evaluator reviews multiple components of this feedback loop: contractual agreements, context evaluation, input evaluation, process evaluation, impact evaluation, effectiveness evaluation, transportability evaluation, sustainability evaluation, and meta-evaluation (Stufflebeam, 2002).

▪ **Logic Models**: display the sequence of actions describing what the program is and the outcomes of the program, as well as how each step is linked to achieve results. Five core components in this depiction of the program action are: inputs, outputs, outcomes, assumptions, and external factors (University of Wisconsin Extension, 2009).

- **Gap Analysis: gap analysis** is a tool for comparing "where we are" to "where we want to be." This method of evaluation comes to education from business and economics, where it has been widely used to compare actual corporate performance with potential performance. The gap in performance is identified and the bridge to improve the gap is defined by performance improvement. This gap is the beginning point for a system-wide improvement process. The gap is seen following the analysis of "where you are" as compared to "where you want to be." This is reflected in a predetermined performance number. The gap analysis can facilitate the improvement process if the users understand the dynamics involved in what created the gaps. The process looks at system problems rather than individual or group shortfalls. Once gaps are identified, then goals and objectives are aligned to create an improvement plan (Dana, 2004).

Today, logic models, gap analysis, management models such as the one designed Stufflebeam, and the work done by Scriven are widely used in nursing education programs in the United States.

Accreditation

The U.S. Department of Education oversees accreditation of schools, colleges, and universities. According to the U.S. Department of Education (2010), "the goal of accreditation is to ensure that education provided by institutions of higher education meets acceptable levels of quality. Accrediting agencies, which are private educational associations of regional or national scope, develop evaluation criteria and conduct peer evaluations to assess whether or not those criteria are met. Institutions and/or programs that request an agency's evaluation and that meet an agency's criteria are then "accredited" by that agency" (para. 2). The goal, stated more basically, is to ensure education provided by higher education institutions meets acceptable levels of quality standards. These standards can be set by regulatory agencies, regional accrediting bodies, and professional accrediting bodies. The outcome for each level of accreditation serves as evidence of a quality unit or institution. Accreditation is important to students, obviously as a sign of quality, but, more important, accreditation is necessary for students attending programs to receive federal dollars to support their education.

Regulatory agencies for nursing programs are generally state nursing boards. The approval obtained by state boards of nursing applies only to the college, school, or department of nursing; this is not an approval process for the entire university or college. State boards of nursing do not directly report to the National Council of State Boards of Nursing (NCSBN), but do fall under the supervision of the state government and, indirectly, the legislature and governor's office. Although state boards are normally closely aligned with the NCSBN, policies, rules, and regulations for schools of nursing seeking state board approval are established by individual state agencies. Approved nursing programs have obtained board of nursing approval through a defined process. This process begins with initial program approval, allowing the program to begin enrollment, and schools follow up with state boards in a process for full approval. Many states require annual reporting by schools of nursing to assure ongoing board of nursing approval. Ongoing program approval requires schools of nursing to meet predetermined benchmarks for National Council Licensure Examination RN Pass Rates, review of a program's Annual Report submitted to the board of nursing, the program's compliance as evaluated with a survey visit if deemed necessary by the state board of nursing, and the program's ongoing compliance with state rules.

Regional accreditation is a continuous improvement process involving the entire university or college. Many of the regional accrediting agencies, such as the Southern Association of Colleges and Schools (SACS), engage the college or university to pursue a continuous improvement process of self-evaluation, reflection, and improvement (SACS, 2010). The SACS is aligned with other regional accrediting bodies. These regional bodies are located in the north-central, western, and northeastern states. All of the regional accrediting agencies subscribe to unifying quality standards for education. One of the best examples of a regional accrediting body is the SACS.

The SACS is a regional body for accrediting of degree-granting higher education institutions in defined southern states. The SACS Commission on Colleges mission "is the enhancement of educational quality throughout the region and it strives to improve the effectiveness of institutions by ensuring that institutions meet standards established by the higher education community that address the needs of society and students" (SACS, 2010, para. 1). The SACS Commission on Colleges accredits associate degree, bachelor's, master's, and doctoral programs in the regionally aligned states. In addition, the SACS accredits some international sites. To meet accreditation standards defined by the SACS Commission, the college or university must comply with the standards established in *Principles of Accreditation: Founda-*

tions for Quality Enhancement and with the policies and procedures of the Commission on Colleges (SACS, 2010).

Accreditation procedures can be found on the regional accrediting websites. The process varies by accrediting body, but all agencies require a self-study or compliance report, which may be followed by a campus visit. The Commission will then review all materials and deny or approve accreditation for a designated time period. All regional accrediting bodies other than the SACS can be found on the website for the Council for Higher Education Accreditation (CHEA) at www .chea.org/Directories/regional.asp Seven regional accrediting bodies are recognized by CHEA.

Professional or national accreditation varies by discipline and is a key to defining a quality unit or discipline within a community college, college, and/or university. For nursing, two widely sought professional accrediting agencies are the National League for Nursing Accrediting Council (NLNAC) and the Commission on Collegiate Nursing Education (CCNE). Both the NLNAC and the CCNE are recognized by the U.S. Department of Education. The CCNE agency accredits only baccalaureate and higher degree programs in nursing. The NLNAC offers accreditation to vocational/ practical nursing programs, associate degree, diploma, and bachelor's, master's, and doctoral programs within nursing schools and/or departments. Seeking accreditation for a school of nursing can be costly regardless of the entity selected for accreditation. Additionally, it should be noted that some schools of nursing select to seek and maintain accreditation from both the NLNAC and the CCNE. For both NLNAC and CCNE accreditation, continuous self-assessment is the key to assuring quality.

NLNAC accreditation provides a nongovernmental approach to recognizing quality in educational programs. Accreditation is a voluntary, self-regulatory process. The accredited institutions have met or exceeded standards identified for quality nursing programs. During the accreditation review, resources invested, processes followed, and results obtained are examined. The NLNAC is also closely tied to state regulatory agency findings related to NCLEX pass rates and licensing rules and regulations (NLNAC, 2002). Standards are well defined and allow schools of nursing to demonstrate quality. Graduation from a school recognized for quality in higher education in the discipline of nursing is required for admission to many graduate programs and for acceptance into many branches of the military.

For NLNAC accreditation, six standards are reviewed in the areas of mission, faculty and staff, curriculum, students, resources, and outcomes. Responses to the standards and sub-standards under each standard are reflected in a report known as the "Self-Study." The

Self-Study affords each school the opportunity to reflect on where it is going, what is in place to achieve the mission and/or what is needed to get there, and what the outcomes are of current efforts. Additionally, a site visit by the NLNAC designated visitors is an important component of the process. Accreditation renewal periods with the NLNAC vary by the findings of the evaluators. The end result of Self-Study is validation of the evidence of delivery of a quality nursing program.

The CCNE is an autonomous agency granting accreditation for baccalaureate, residency, and higher degree programs for validation of quality and integrity. The global mission of the CCNE is to protect the public health (CCNE, 2009). This is also a voluntary, self-regulatory process for recognizing effective educational practices in nursing education. For CCNE accreditation, four standards are reviewed in the school's self-assessment. These standards are: Mission and Governance, Institutional Commitment and Resources, Curriculum and Teaching-Learning Practices, and Aggregate Student and Faculty Outcomes. The first three standards speak to program quality and the last standard assures program effectiveness. CCNE accreditation can be given to a school of nursing for up to 10 years. Like the Self-Study, the Self-Assessment yields evidence for validation of a quality nursing program.

Program Evaluation

Program evaluation is an ongoing process in nursing education and requires a framework for evaluation to be adopted by the faculty, standards and outcomes to be defined, as well as a timeline for measurement of achievement. Program evaluation focuses on review and improvement. The need for curriculum revision, resources, and faculty and staff may become apparent during this ongoing review process.

Program evaluation allows educators to facilitate meaningful change while providing feedback. Evaluation is an ongoing process included in all program development stages. There are six general evaluation frameworks:

- Objectives-oriented: measures attainment of identified goals and objectives.
- Management-oriented: gathers data for managerial decisions as a source of evaluation.
- Consumer-oriented: uses the voice of the consumer to evaluate the curricula and instructional products.

▓ Expertise-oriented: expert evaluates the quality of the educational program.
▓ Adversary-oriented: opposing points of view of different evaluators (pro and con) are the central point of the evaluation.
▓ Naturalistic- and participant-oriented: focusing on naturalistic inquiry and involvement of participants (stakeholders are a part of what is being evaluated) is central in determining needs, data collected, and outcomes of the evaluation. (Welch & Reineke, 2003)

Whether you select a framework for evaluation focused on attainment of objectives or a management-oriented framework, all program evaluation gathers evidence for measurement against predetermined outcomes. The framework will provide the steps to outcome attainment. All program evaluation should be systematic and ongoing to be effective. With systematic program evaluation, decisions are based on the evidence rather than assumptions. Program evaluation should have utility; that is, stakeholders should be identified, credible evaluators should be enlisted in the process, appropriate questions and answers should be asked and sought, values should be clarified, the reporting system should be clear, and reporting and dissemination of findings should be timely to obtain the impact or feedback from the evaluation (Centers for Disease Control and Prevention [CDC], 2004). How did the findings of this program evaluation result in changes in the program? Additionally, frameworks for program evaluation should be feasible and reveal and display accurate information. Steps described in a general program evaluation process reflect engaging stakeholders, describing the program, focusing on the evaluation design, gathering credible evidence, justifying conclusions against standards, and providing feedback on findings and lessons learned for stakeholders (CDC, 2004).

Course Evaluation

According to Oermann et al. (2009a), "planning for assessment at the course level provides an opportunity for faculty to ensure that their methods collect the information they need, are fair, are used consistently by the teachers and preceptors in that course, and reflect the standards set by faculty" (p. 276). Course evaluations are frequently viewed as stressful and challenging. At times, faculty members question the advantage of having the course evaluation. Though they understand that course evaluations are mandated by accrediting agencies, state boards of nursing, and the institutions, the applicability of the evaluation tends to be the aspect that is questioned. Lowenstein and Bradshaw (2004) stated that evaluations are to be performed to provide the foundation for making decisions about the course and/ or other aspects related to the course. Because the process is driven by these other entities, the functionality of the course evaluations for the course is frequently questioned by the faculty members involved in the course. What aspects are included on the evaluation? When is the evaluation scheduled to be completed? Is the participation in the evaluation process coerced in some manner? What impact does the course evaluation have on the individual faculty member? So many questions are raised by the process of course evaluations.

As the process of course evaluation and EBT are considered, minimal research evidence can be found related to course evaluation. Textbooks and manuscripts speak to the process and current status of course evaluations but research evidence is not readily accessible. As a result, the evidence to be used falls in the areas of opinions, current practices, and accepted processes.

Sewell, Culpa-Bondal, and Colvin (2008) provide an overview of the current practices viewed within the evaluation process. The determination of the evaluation process is based upon the faculty members structuring each course syllabus to concentrate on the program objectives. This structuring or mapping process challenges the strengths and weaknesses perceived in each course and across the curriculum. By ascertaining the linkages between the course syllabus, program objectives, and the total curriculum, a systematic course analysis process can be established. Sewell et al. (2008) state that "support for the scholarship of teaching and learning by academic leadership is crucial to a successful program outcome process" (p. 100S). By identifying the "data-drive incremental multidimensional processes and procedures that positively impact the teaching and learning process" (Sewell et al., 2008, p. 100S), the faculty members can formulate an effective and useful evaluation process. Most of the literature notes two types of course evaluation processes: formative and summative evaluation processes.

Formative evaluation is "the gathering of data to make decisions during the planning, development, and implementation of the program" (Lowenstein & Bradshaw, 2004, p. 353). Other terms used for this type of evaluation are content or process evaluation. Formative evaluation is viewed as the ongoing, periodical, and routinely done assessment of the progression of the course process (Caputi, 2010; Lowenstein & Bradshaw, 2004). This type of evaluation can take many different forms. Faculty members tend to use this type of assessment to get at the essences of quality of the course. It can be done through the use of 1-minute papers, as noted in Chapter 6, which ask the students what key item (or items) was effectively covered during a session of the course. A similar formative evaluation is the muddiest point assignment, also discussed in Chapter 6, which allows the student to list any areas from the content presented that continue to be confusing. Formative evaluations can also be surveys given at key times within the semester to assess the students' perception of the course. According to Caputi (2010), "the purpose of this type of evaluation is to improve the instruction as the course is progressing to ensure students are learning before the end of the term when it is too late to make adjustments" (p. 43). When seeking formative evaluative information, the faculty member initially determines the impetus and stimulus for the data collection process. The questions and/or other data collecting methods can then converge on gathering the appropriate material being sought.

At times, the formative evaluations could be directed toward the determination of the appropriateness and/or success of a new teaching strategy. On other occasions, the focus for the evaluation could be on the coverage of the content needed within the course. Thus, formative evaluations should be done at intervals and with a purpose. Oermann et al. (2009b) view formative evaluation as an educative process that is directed toward supplying "feedback to students about their strengths and weaknesses and to identify strategies to address both" (p. 353). Within formative evaluation, the focus is directed toward the student and assisting the student to be successful in the course. Every effort is used to ensure that appropriate teaching strategies are used to substantiate the effective coverage of the material selected to be addressed within the learning process.

According to Bastable (2003), "the purpose of process or formative evaluation is to make adjustments in an educational activity as soon as they are needed, whether those adjustments be in personnel, materials, facilitates, learning objectives, or even one's own attitude" (p. 496). The adjustments need to be viewed as an ongoing course of action to confirm that every aspect of the course is functioning in an appropriate manner. By using this type of evaluation effectively, the faculty member can make changes as needed within the course prior to a negative outcome for the student cohort. Because each student cohort has unique needs and learning expectations, the use of formative evaluation allows for the changes to be made that are appropriate for each student cohort. Does that mean that the faculty member needs to be querying the students and changing directions every week? No. It does mean that at intervals, the learning environment should be challenged to verify that the needs of all those involved in the learning are being addressed.

Bastable (2003) establishes that "learner behavior, teacher behavior, learner-teacher interaction, learner response to teaching material and methods, and characteristics of the environment are all aspects of the learning experience within the scope of process evaluation"

(p. 497). Because formative evaluations are designed to look at the content and/or purpose, each of these areas needs to be authenticated as effective.

Summative evaluations (also called outcome evaluations) are "done at the end of a semester or course to provide the final judgment as to whether or not the student has achieved the educational goals, in effect judging if the student's practice meets established standards of safety and competence" (Oermann et al., 2009b, p. 353). Summative evaluations are used to confirm the overall success of the course, not the individual aspects within the course. Frequently, this evaluation process is uniform for all courses and all programs within the school and university. As a result, the information gained from these summative (outcome) evaluations is based on the content that is general and applicable across courses, programs, and schools. The questions habitually are global in nature. Thus, the applications for modifying individual courses are less apparent.

In addition to the end of course surveys that are provided and controlled by the school, another example of summative evaluations is the final examination used within a course. Caputi (2010) suggests that "the information from the summative evaluation is used not only to assign a grade to the student's performance, but also to revise and refine the course—making it better for future students" (p. 43). The final assignments within any course are used to determine the success of the course. From these final assignments (such as final examinations or formal papers), the students' performance can be viewed. By examining the course grade analysis, changes can be determined to improve the course.

Evaluations are a key part within the educational environment. As faculty members consider the different aspects of this process, the anticipated function of the process and the methods for utilizing the information acquired need to be carefully and thoughtfully considered. Bastable (2003) makes a sound recommendation when stating that "evaluation as an afterthought is, at best, a poor idea and, at worst, a dangerous one" (p. 494). The entire evaluation flow must be carefully determined as the program is developed, not left to be an afterthought. By painstakingly and meticulously determining the multidimensional aspects imperative to a beneficial evaluation, the results found through the appraisal process can be analyzed and utilized to improve the learning environment. According to Lowenstein and Bradshaw (2004), intrinsic in the definition of evaluation "is the understanding that results of the evaluation will be used to provide feedback concerning teaching for the development of faculty and refinement of teaching skills" (p. 363). If the resulting information cannot be or is not used to improve the program, course, or methods of the faculty member, it needs to be reviewed and revised. Material not used in this nature is inconsequential to the learning environment. Each piece of data collected should be utilized to move the program forward to the educational goals set by the faculty within the school's mission statement and program objectives.

Within many programs of education, the gap analysis process is used to analyze and organize the results found through the summative end-of-course evaluations. According to the Business Dictionary (2010), a gap analysis is a "technique for determining the steps to be taken in moving from a current state to a desired future state" (lines 1–2). A gap analysis strives to identify two key levels of factors, such as the current understanding held by students and the desired understanding wanted by students. From these two levels, the differences between the two levels are determined, which is viewed as the gap. In the process of collecting and determining the gap analysis, the present and future states are both sought. By comparing the two levels, a determination of what areas need to be addressed in the process can be identified. Schools that employ the gap analysis process for summative evaluation establish the benchmark level that is acceptable for the gap analysis values. Areas in the course that do not meet this benchmark are then expected to be addressed prior to future provisions of that course. If all areas of the summative evaluations meet or exceed the benchmark level established, the faculty member and/or team can feel confident that the course is meeting the needs of the school based on the areas covered within the summative evaluation. Faculty members must carefully examine the outcomes from the gap analysis. For all areas denoted within the analysis, any sporadic events or evidence of a pattern evident in more than one semester must be included in the interpretation of the results.

Faculty Evaluation

Though summative and formative evaluations include assessment of the faculty member in the process, the faculty member also participates in a separate evaluation process related to the total role of the faculty member. According to McKay (2008), "every teacher has to live with the basics of what accountants call 'counting the beans' in using evaluation to check the bottom line on planned outcomes" (p. 258). The job descriptions, tenure/promotion criteria, and accreditation standards provide the framework that guides the faculty evaluation. Job descriptions are established by the institution to reflect the overall teaching and clinical responsibilities in addition to the general faculty participatory expectations such as committee work, scholarly endeavors, and research/practice undertakings. For most institutions, the faculty members are obliged to document their different activities reflective of the aspects listed on the job descriptions. Commonly, faculty members are asked to establish annual performance goals that indicate those areas on which they anticipate focusing during the upcoming academic year. These annual goals are then used to drive the yearly performance evaluation. One strategy for faculty to use when establishing the annual goals is to investigate which tenure and/or promotion criteria are appropriate to concentrate on for this year. When faculty member use the different criteria established within the tenure and/or promotion guidelines as their annual goals, they receive double "bang for their buck." It meets the annual goal expectations for advancement while moving the faculty member closer to being ready to seek promotion and/or tenure. The guidelines provided in the tenure and promotion documents along with the materials found included on the job description give a clear picture of the institution's expectations for faculty members. These annual goals developed by the individual faculty member are usually reviewed and approved by some member of the administration within the school. That person could be a chairperson, associate dean, faculty development designee, or dean-appointed representative or dean. The review of the goals is done to ensure that faculty members are continuing to grow and develop in the role of academician. Once the faculty member has launched the annual goals, a mechanism and/or strategy needs to be established to assemble the needed documents. Throughout the year, the faculty member needs to have a place to put any documents that will be used during the annual evaluation to support the successful completion of the designated goals.

The work documented by Hessler and Humphreys (2008) is directed toward the effective use of student evaluations, particularly by novice faculty. The information provided can be used by all levels of faculty members as they deal with the comments submitted by students. According to Hessler and Humphreys (2008), "students can provide valuable feedback on instructional techniques and course design but cannot necessarily judge whether the material in the course is current or whether the instructors knows the subject matter" (p. 187). Having an understanding concerning the focus of student evaluations helps faculty members recognize how the material can be used to strengthen skills and applications within the faculty role and the classroom (see **Table 9-1**). According to Hessler and Humphreys (2008), studies have found that the grade expected in the course might or might not have a bearing on the outcomes of the evaluation. In one research study they reviewed, it was found that lower expected grades = lower evaluations. But in another study, the opposite was true—lower expected grades did not correlate to poorer evaluations. Fairness by the faculty along with a perceived availability of the faculty member frequently results in faculty evaluations that reflect the actual

Table 9-1

Suggestions for Improving Student Evaluation Response Rates

- Arrange evaluations to be accomplished at times when final examinations are not planned or scheduled.
- Make sure that students have ample time to complete the evaluation forms.
- Take the time to explain the evaluation process prior to administering the forms.
- As explanations for the evaluation process are provided, ensure that students understand who or what they are to evaluate—course, faculty, curriculum, clinical, etc.
- Clarify the importance and value of comments—both positive and negative in nature—for the improvement of the program.
- Encourage students to provide specific examples related to negative comments and suggestions for improving the course.
- Remember that the student is the consumer of the educational experience.
- Validate that the evaluation tool addresses the aspects that are key to improving the course and/ or faculty.
- Work to ensure that the tool is not so global that specific areas of improvement become hard to identify.

Source: Adapted from Hessler, K., & Humphreys, J. (2008). Student evaluations: Advice for novice faculty. *Journal of Nursing Education, 47*(4), 188.

Table 9-2

Recommendations for Faculty to Use When Considering Student Evaluations

- Use the expertise of seasoned faculty at intervals to validate the information documented within student evaluations.
- When using a seasoned faculty member to evaluate teaching abilities, identify key goals for the individual to focus on to guide the comments and recommendations.
- At different times, take advantage of sitting in on proficient faculty members as they conduct the classroom and/or clinical experience.
- Select and utilize at least one faculty mentor.
- Trend the student evaluation data instead of dwelling on one cohort's comments. Trends are key to identifying areas needing improvement.
- Utilize formative summaries to provide a more rounded evaluation of the learning environment instead of depending on one summative evaluation.
- Maintain an open mind and willingness to strive to improve on what is currently used and to incorporate new teaching methods as needed. Don't become stale in your teaching.

Source: Adapted from Hessler, K. & Humphreys, J. (2008). Student evaluations: Advice for novice faculty. *Journal of Nursing Education, 47*(4), 188.

activities occurring in the classroom instead of the entirety of the interaction with a faculty member (see **Table 9-2**). Although the original purpose for asking for student evaluations was to improve the course delivery and teaching environment, schools have begun to use these evaluations during the annual faculty evaluations and tenure/ promotion processes. The summative evaluations developed by the school/university do not address the key component reflected in the job descriptions and the tenure/promotion guidelines. Hessler and Humphreys (2008) raise the concern that the reliability and validity of the student evaluations are not conclusively proven. Yet, they do remain an important aspect within the evaluation process. Another grave aspect that must be considered in relation to these evaluations is the timing of them and any coercion that might be evident. When students are forced to complete the evaluations in order to receive conclusion to the course, the resulting evaluation results are tainted. Questions must be raised in these situations as to the appropriateness of any results when the results were forced. Care must be given to encouraging the completion of student evaluation without the use of threats.

Summary Thoughts

Evidence-based evaluation involves many components. By determining the model or framework you would like to use for evaluation, directions for evidence obtainment are identified. All stakeholders must understand and be committed to the model used for evaluation for the data gathered for evidence to be valid, reliable, and, most important, meaningful. Although accreditation assures program quality and requires in-depth self-appraisal or self-evaluation, program evaluation should be in place and continuous to ensure program purposes and standards are being met.

Summary Points

1. Because evaluation is a crucial aspect of education, it must be carefully and thoroughly discussed and incorporated into the process of evidence-based teaching.
2. Evaluation has an impact on every aspect within the educational process.
3. The process of systematically collecting, analyzing, and interpreting data to aid in the determination of quality educational outcomes is crucial for the establishment and management of effective nursing programs.
4. Accreditation agencies mandate that each facet of a program be carefully, methodically, and logically appraised to reflect the quality of the programmatic goals and outcomes designated within the program.
5. Although faculty members understand that course evaluations are mandated by accrediting agencies, state boards of nursing, and the employing institutions, the applicability of the evaluation tends to be the aspect that is questioned.
6. Textbooks and manuscripts note the process and current status of course evaluations, but research evidence is not readily accessible.

7. By ascertaining the linkages between each course syllabus, program objectives, and the total curriculum, a systematic course analysis process can be established.

8. Formative evaluation is viewed as the ongoing, periodical, and routinely done assessment of the progression of the course process.

9. When seeking formative evaluative information, the faculty member initially determines the impetus and stimulus for the data collection process.

10. Within formative evaluation, the focus is directed toward the student and assisting the student to be successful in the course.

11. The learning environment should be challenged to verify that the needs of all those involved in the learning are being addressed.

12. Summative evaluations are used to confirm the overall success of the course, not the individual aspects within the course.

13. The information gained from summative (outcome) evaluations is based on the content that is general and applicable across courses, programs, and schools.

14. The entire evaluation flow must be carefully determined as the program is developed, not left to be an afterthought.

15. Each piece of data collected should be utilized to move the program forward to the educational goals set by the faculty within the school's mission statement and program objectives.

16. A gap analysis strives to identify two key levels of factors, such as the current understanding held by students and the desired understanding wanted by students.

17. Areas in the course that do not meet this benchmark are then expected to be addressed prior to future provisions of that course. If all areas of the summative evaluations meet or exceed the benchmark level established, the faculty member and/or team can feel confident that the course is meeting the needs of the school based on the areas covered within the summative evaluation.

18. Though summative and formative evaluations include assessment of the faculty members in the process, the faculty member also participates in a separate evaluation process related to the total role of the faculty member.

19. Commonly, faculty members are asked to establish annual performance goals that indicate those areas on which they anticipate focusing during the upcoming academic year.

20. Having an understanding concerning the focus of student evaluations helps faculty members recognize how the material can be used to strengthen skills and applications within the faculty role and the classroom.

21. Evaluation provides the evidence needed for delivering effective teaching methodologies, setting appropriate curricula, and directing program development.

22. Evaluation models are used to help define the characteristics or features of an evaluation, what concepts to study, and the processes or methods needed to extract critical data, evidence, and outcomes.

23. Today, logic models, gap analysis, management models such as the one designed by Stufflebeam, and the work done by Scriven are widely used in nursing education programs in the United States.

24. Accrediting agencies are monitored by the Department of Education. Accreditation can be regional, such as SACS accreditation, or professional/ national, such as NLNAC and/or CCNE accreditation. Regulatory agencies such as state boards of nursing also provide program approval.

25. Program evaluation is an ongoing process in nursing education and requires a framework for evaluation to be adopted by the faculty, standards and outcomes to be defined, as well as a timeline for measurement of achievement to be set. Program evaluation focuses on review and improvement.

Tips for Nurse Educators to Use

1. Once the faculty member has launched the annual goals, a mechanism and/or strategy needs to be established to assemble the needed documents.

2. When faculty members use the different criteria established within the tenure and/or promotion guidelines as their annual goals, it meets the annual goal expectations for advancement while moving faculty members closer to being ready to seek promotion and/or tenure.

3. The review of the goals is done to ensure that faculty members are continuing to grow and develop in the role of academician.

4. Throughout the year, the faculty member needs to have a place to file any documents that will be used during the annual evaluation to support the successful completion of the designated goals.

5. Fairness by the faculty along with a perceived availability of the faculty member frequently results in faculty evaluations that reflect the nature presented in the classroom.

6. Care must be given to encouraging the completion of student evaluations without the use of threats.

7. Evaluation provides the evidence needed for delivering effective teaching methodologies, curricula, and program development. Therefore, it is very important that each faculty member buy into the model selected for the nursing unit to use for evaluation.

8. Accreditation can be very costly. Planning for accreditation costs in the annual budget is a very important step for nursing education administrators.

9. Accreditation may have hidden costs, such as the need for outside consultants during the self-study or appraisal process.

10. Some states are now recognizing national/professional accreditation and are not requiring state boards of nursing to make annual site visits or annual reports to the state board of nursing. Check with your state board of nursing to see if this may be the case in your state.

11. Use the self-study/self-appraisal process to recognize the strengths of your program, and realize that this is also a very important time to gather data needed to share with college or university administration about needed resources such as technology, space, or salary alignment for the nursing unit.

References

Bastable, S. B. (2003). *Nurse as educator: Principles of teaching and learning for nursing practice* (2nd ed.). Sudbury, MA: Jones and Bartlett Publishers.

Bruce, B. C., & Rubin, A. (1993). *Electronic quills: A situated evaluation of using computers for writing in classrooms*. Hillsdale, NJ: Lawrence Erlbaum Associates.

Business Dictionary. (2010). Definition—gap analysis. Retrieved January 18, 2010, from www.businessdictionary.com/definition/gap-analysis.html

Caputi, L. (2010). An overview of the educational process. In L. Caputi (Ed.), *Teaching nursing: The art and science* (2nd ed., pp. 27–47).

Commission on Collegiate Nursing Education (CCNE). (2009). CCNE mission statement and goals. Retrieved March 23, 2010, from http://www.aacn.nche.edu/accreditation/mission.htm

Centers for Disease Control and Prevention. (2004). CDC evaluation working group. Retrieved March 23, 2010, from http://www.cdc.gov/eval/standard.htm

Dana, C. (2004). Gap analysis: Overview of identifying gaps process. Middle Level School Principal Seminar, March 30, 2004 Austin, Texas. Retrieved March 23, 2010, from http://www.utdanacenter.org/downloads/presentations/gapanalysis_march04.pdf

Eisener, E. W. (1976). Education connoisseurship and criticism: Their forms and Functions in educational evaluation. *Journal of Aesthetic Education, 10,* 135–150.

Hessler, K., & Humphreys, J. (2008). Student evaluations: Advice for novice faculty. *Journal of Nursing Education, 47*(4), 187–189.

Kirkpatrick, D. L. (1998). *Evaluating training programs: The four levels* (2nd ed.). San Francisco, CA: Berrett-Koehler Publishers.

Lowenstein, A. J., & Bradshaw, M. J. (2004). *Fuszard's innovative teaching strategies in nursing* (3rd ed.). Sudbury, MA: Jones and Bartlett Publishers.

McKay, J. (2008). Evaluating teaching and learning. In B. Penn (Ed.), *Mastering the teaching role: A guide for nurse educators* (pp. 255–264).

National League of Nursing Accrediting Commission, Inc. (2002). NLNAC mission. Retrieved March 23, 2010, from http://www.nlnac.org/About%20NLNAC/AboutNLNAC.htm#MISSION

Newhouse, R. P., & Johnson, K. (2009). A case study in evaluating infrastructure for EBP and selecting a model. *Journal of Nursing Administration, 39*(10), 409–411.

Oermann, M. H., Saewert, K. J., Charasika, M., & Yarbrough, S. S. (2009a). Assessment and grading practices in schools of nursing: National survey findings part I. *Nursing Education Perspectives, 30*(5), 274–278.

Oermann, M. H., Saewert, K. J., Charasika, M., & Yarbrough, S. S. (2009b). Assessment and grading practices in schools of nursing: National survey findings part II. *Nursing Education Perspectives, 30*(6), 352–357.

Scriven, M. (1972). Pros and cons of goal-free evaluation. *Evaluation Comment, 3*(4), 1–7.

Sewell, J., Culpa-Bondal, F., & Colvin, M. (2008). Nursing program assessment and evaluation: Evidence-based decision making improves outcomes. *CIN: Computers, Informatics, Nursing,* 98S–101S.

Southern Association of Colleges and Schools (SACS). (2010.) Accrediting standards. Retrieved March 3, 2010, from http://www.sacscoc.org/index.asp

Stufflebeam, D. L. (2002). The CIPP model for evaluation. In D. L. Stufflebeam & T. Kellaghan (Eds.), *The international handbook of educational evaluation* (Chapter 2). Boston, MA: Kluwer Academic Publishers.

Stufflebeam, D. L., Madaus, G. F., & Kellaghan, T. (2000). *Evaluation models: Viewpoints on educational and human services evaluation* (2nd ed.). Boston, MA: Kluwer Academic Publishers.

Tyler, R. W. (1949). *Basic principles of curriculum and instruction.* Chicago, IL: The University of Chicago Press.

University of Wisconsin Extension. (2009). Program development and evaluation. Retrieved March 12, 2010, from http://www.uwex.edu/ces/pdande/evaluation/evallogicmodel.html

U.S. Department of Education. (2010). The U.S. Department of Education database of accredited postsecondary institutions and programs. Retrieved April 2, 2010, from http://ope.ed.gov/accreditation/index.aspx

Virginia Tech. (2009). Design shop: Lessons in effective teaching. Retrieved March 12, 2010, from http://www.edtech.vt.edu/edtech/id/eval/eval.html

Welch, W., & Reineke, R. A. (2003). *National Visiting Committee (NVC) handbook.* Kalamazoo, MI: Western Michigan University, The Evaluation Center.

Worthen, B. R., Sanders, J. R., & Fitzpatrick. (1997). *Program evaluation: Alternative approaches and practical guidelines* (2nd ed.). New York, NY: Longman.

Web Links

A list of accredited post secondary higher education programs is available at http:// ope.ed.gov/accreditation.

View the National Council of State Boards of Nursing home page at www.ncsbn.org/ index.htm.

View the Southern Regional Education Board home page at www.sreb.org.

View the Southern Association of Colleges and Schools home page at www.sacs.org.

View the Council for Higher Education Accreditation home page at www.chea.org/ Directories/regional.asp.

View the National League of Nursing Accrediting Commission, Inc. home page at www.nlnac.org.

View the Commission on Collegiate Nursing Education (CCNE) home page at www .aacn.nche.edu/Accreditation/index.htm.

Multiple Choice Questions

1. Individuals working in an institution of higher education who need to be evaluated to ensure a quality program of study are the:

   A. administration, faculty, and students.
   B. faculty only.
   C. students only.
   D. administration and students only.

Rationale:

Within this process, administration, faculty, curriculum, and students are all assessed to determine their unique parts within the advancement of a quality program of study resulting in highly qualified students ready to assume the role of competent entry-level registered nurse.

2. During the establishment of the evaluation process, faculty members work to structure the:

   A. course expectations to the course objectives.
   B. each individual syllabus to the program objectives.
   C. course philosophy to the program mission.
   D. course objectives to the program objectives.

Rationale:

The determination of the evaluation process is based upon the faculty members structuring their syllabi to concentrate on the program objectives. This structuring or mapping process challenges the strengths and weaknesses perceived in each course and across the curriculum.

3. A systematic course analysis process can be established when a linkage is noted between

   A. total curriculum and school mission.
   B. the course syllabus, program objectives, and the total curriculum.
   C. total curriculum and faculty job descriptions.
   D. each individual syllabus, faculty job descriptions, and the school mission.

Rationale:

By ascertaining the linkages between each individual syllabus, program objectives, and the total curriculum, a systematic course analysis process can be established. Sewell et al. (2008) state that "support for the scholarship of teaching and learning by academic leadership is crucial to a successful program outcome process" (p. 100S). By identifying the "data-driven incremental multidimensional processes and procedures that positively impact the teaching and learning process" (Sewell et al., p. 100S), the faculty members can formulate an effective and useful evaluation process.

4. Formative evaluations strive to gather data to make decisions during the
   A. planning and development stages of the curriculum.
   B. planning stage only.
   C. implementation stage only.
   D. planning, development, and implementation stages.

Rationale:

Formative evaluation is "the gathering of data to make decisions during the planning, development, and implementation of the program" (Lowenstein & Bradshaw, 2004, p. 353).

5. Formative evaluation us viewed as

   A. **the ongoing, periodical, and routinely done assessment of the progression of the course process.**
   B. a single episode of the progression of the course process.
   C. the final assessment of the progression of the course process.
   D. an evaluation of the faculty member only.

Rationale:

Formative evaluation is viewed as the ongoing, periodical, and routinely done assessment of the progression of the course process (Caputi, 2010; Lowenstein & Bradshaw, 2004). This type of evaluation can take many different forms. Faculty members tend to use this type of assessment to determine the quality of the course.

6. When seeking formative evaluation information, faculty members need to carefully determine
   A. the student cohort makeup.
   B. **the specific reasons for the evaluation.**
   C. which faculty member is to be evaluated.
   D. only how to collect the data.

Rationale:

When seeking formative evaluative information, the faculty member initially determines the impetus and stimulus for the data collection process. The questions and/or other data collecting methods can then converge on gathering the appropriate material being sought.

7. Summative evaluations are set up to
   A. cover the same materials as found in the formative evaluations.
   B. provide a summarization of the material identified in the formative evaluations.
   C. **uniformly evaluate all courses and all programs within the school and university.**
   D. carefully collect data on courses and programs within the school.

Rationale:

Summative evaluations are used to confirm the overall success of the course, not the individual aspects within the course. Frequently, this evaluation process is uniform for all courses and all programs within the school and university. As a result, the information gained from these summative (outcome) evaluations is based on the content that is general and applicable across courses, programs, and schools. The questions habitually are global in nature.

8. The guiding documents that provide the framework for the annual evaluation of faculty members are
    A. course evaluations and job descriptions.
    B. summative evaluations, formative evaluations, and gap analysis.
    C. job descriptions and accreditation standards.
    D. job descriptions, tenure/promotion criteria, and accreditation standards.

Rationale:

The job descriptions, tenure/promotion criteria, and accreditation standards provide the framework that guides the faculty evaluation. Job descriptions are established by the institution to reflect the overall teaching and clinical responsibilities in addition to the general faculty participatory expectations, such as committee work, scholarly endeavors, and research/practice undertakings. For most institutions, the faculty members are obliged to document their different activities reflective of the aspects listed on the job descriptions.

9. Faculty members often are expected to develop annual professional goals to strive to meet; these goals are validated by:
    A. the dean of the school of nursing.
    B. the faculty member only
    C. the chairperson, associate dean, or dean-appointed representative.
    D. both the chairperson and the dean of the school of nursing.

Rationale:

The annual goals developed by the individual faculty member are usually reviewed and approved by some member of the administration within the school. That person could be a chairperson, associate dean, faculty development designee, or dean-appointed representative. The review of the goals is done to ensure that faculty members are continuing to grow and develop in the role of academician.

10. Regional accreditation differs from professional or national accreditation in that
    A. regional accreditation is voluntary.
    B. professional or national accreditation is voluntary.

    C. **regional accreditation applies to an entire institution**.

    D.   professional or national accreditation applies to an entire institution.

Rationale:

All accreditation is voluntary, and only regional accreditation is sought by the entire institution. Professional or national accreditation is sought by individual professional schools within the institution.

11. Program evaluation can be described as a(n)

    A.   cyclic activity done before accreditation or re-affirmation.

    B. **continuous activity done to fulfill program purposes**.

    C.   activity done in isolation of state standards.

    D.   activity done in isolation of national standards.

Rationale:

Program evaluation is a continuous activity undertaken to fulfill the program purposes. If evaluation only occurs during a self-study, indicators occurring in the years between accreditation may not be examined. All program evaluation occurs in light of current state and national standards set within the discipline or profession.

12. Five core components in the depiction of the logic model for evaluation are

    A. **inputs, outputs, outcomes, assumptions, and external factors**.

    B.   Contractual Agreements, Context Evaluation, Input Evaluation, Process Evaluation, and Impact Evaluation.

    C.   Impact Evaluation, Effectiveness Evaluation, Transportability Evaluation, Sustainability Evaluation, and Meta-evaluation.

    D.   inputs, outputs, effectiveness, assumptions, and external factors.

Rationale:

The core components of the logic model are inputs, outputs, outcomes, assumptions, and external factors for program evaluation. Options b and c are components of Stufflebeam's CIPP model, and option d is a combination of the logic and CIPP models.

13. Gap analysis can facilitate the improvement process if the user understands that the "gap" is

    A.   seen following the analysis of "where you want to be" and "where you have been."

    B.   a real-time picture of where you want to be in the future.

    C.   the analysis of national indicators and where you are in comparison to these indicators.

    D. **following the analysis of "where you are" as compared to "where you want to be."**

Rationale:

The gap analysis can facilitate the improvement process if the users understand the dynamics involved in what created the gaps. Therefore, where you are as compared to where you want to be in the correct choice. Option a is not of importance, as the past will not aid in finding the gap. Options b and c are not plausible, as gap analysis is the gap in individual performance that is identified and the bridge to improve the gap is defined by performance improvement.

14. Schools of nursing may select to seek accreditation from the Commission on Collegiate Nursing Education (CCNE) rather than the National League for Nursing Accrediting Council (NLNAC) because

   A. the CCNE is accredited by the Department of Education.
   B. the CCNE accredits residency programs.
   C. the NLNAC does not accredit higher degree programs.
   D. the NLNAC is not accredited by the Department of Education.

Rationale:

Both the CCNE and the NLNAC are accredited by the Department of Education. Both the CCNE and the NLNAC accredit higher degree programs. Option b is correct, as the CCNE also accredits residency programs.

Discussion Questions

1. What types of course evaluations have you been involved with in the past either as a student or as a faculty member? Think carefully about what you consider as the strengths and challenges of using those types of course evaluations to improve the delivery of a course. What would you change to improve the process?

Considerations:

Formative evaluation is "the gathering of data to make decisions during the planning, development, and implementation of the program" (Lowenstein & Bradshaw, 2004, p. 353). Other terms used for this type of evaluation are content or process evaluation. Formative evaluation is viewed as the ongoing, periodical, and routinely done assessment of the progression of the course process (Caputi, 2010; Lowenstein & Bradshaw, 2004). This type of evaluation can take many different venues. Faculty members tend to use this form to get at the essences of quality of the course. Summative evaluations (also called outcome evaluations) are "done at the end of a semester or course to provide the final judgment as to whether or not the student has achieved the educational goals, in effect judging if the student's practice meets established standards of safety and competence" (Oermann et al., 2009b, p. 353). Summative evaluations are used to confirm the overall success of the course, not the individual aspects within the course. Frequently, this evaluation process is uniform for all courses and all programs within the school and university. As a result, the information gained from these summative (outcome) evaluations is based on the content that is general and applicable across courses, programs, and schools.

2. Do you think schools should seek both professional program accreditation and regional accreditation? Please provide a rationale for your answer.

Considerations:

Graduation from an accredited program fully recognized by a national professional association such as the NLNAC or the CCNE is required for students to progress to military service and graduate education. Additionally, professional accreditation is required by some state boards of nursing and many state higher education coordinating boards. There is a trend currently for state boards of nursing to waive campus visits in states where this is required if the school of nursing has full professional accreditation from the NLNAC or the CCNE. While the institution seeks overall university or college quality recognition through regional accrediting agencies such as the SACS, professional accreditation for any practice discipline assures the public of the quality of individual school, college, or departmental educational practices.

3. Because performance evaluations are key to helping each of us to improve, what aspects would seem best to evaluate? How does a department and/ or faculty member reflect these areas to demonstrate competency of the skills?

Considerations:

See Tables 9-1 and 9-2 for areas to consider for improving personal performance aspects. The job descriptions, tenure/promotion criteria, and accreditation standards provide the framework that guides the faculty evaluation. Job descriptions are established by the institution to reflect the overall teaching and clinical responsibilities in addition to the general faculty participatory expectations, such as committee work, scholarly endeavors, and research/practice undertakings. For most institutions, the faculty members are obliged to document their different activities reflective of the aspects listed on the job descriptions.

Teaching Scenario

1. Invite the students to perform a brief mock accreditation review of a nursing program, either the program where they are currently enrolled or a neighboring program. Refer the students to the following website, where they may explore the components evaluated in the accreditation process: www.aacn.nche.edu/Accreditation/pdf/standards09.pdf.

2. Explore the current evaluation plan used in your program. The students may decide what type of evaluation plan is being used and how the feedback loop in this program works to enhance program delivery. The students may want to attend school of nursing evaluation committee meetings or interview the faculty member who leads evaluation in this program.

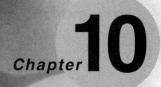

Chapter **10**

Competency and Certification

Linda Caputi

Chapter Objectives

At the conclusion of the chapter, the learner will be able to:

1. Discuss the process used by the National League for Nursing to establish the Certified Nurse Educator (CNE) program.
2. State the items included within the CNE test blueprint.
3. Explain the different aspects involved in the determination of competencies.
4. List the steps needed to prepare to take the CNE examination.
5. Discuss the impact that certification has on a profession.

Key Terms

➤ American Nurses Credentialing Center (ANCC)

➤ Certification

➤ Certified Nurse Educator (CNE)

➤ Competency

➤ Feasibility study

➤ National Commission for Certifying Agencies (NCCA)

➤ National Council of State Boards of Nursing (NCSBN)

- ➤ National League for Nursing Accrediting Commission (NLNAC)
- ➤ Needs assessment
- ➤ Nurse educator competencies
- ➤ Practice analysis
- ➤ Scope of practice
- ➤ Staff development
- ➤ Test blueprint
- ➤ Think tank

Introduction

The notion of evidence-based teaching is influencing faculty from many vantage points. For example, the **National Council of State Boards of Nursing (NCSBN)** has published a position paper "Evidence-Based Nursing Education for Regulation." The NCSBN looked at which teaching methodologies had the best student outcomes (Spector, 2006). The NCSBN's recommendations for evidence-based nursing education for regulation include teaching methods, assimilation of the students into the role of nursing, promoting faculty–student relationships, and other areas of teaching.

Furthermore, the new 2008 Standards for accreditation of nursing programs by the **National League for Nursing Accrediting Commission (NLNAC)** also address evidence-based teaching. Criterion 2.5 states, "Faculty performance reflects scholarship and evidence-based practice" (NLNAC, 2008, p. 64). This is a criterion for all levels of nursing education. But if the NLNAC defines evidence-based practice as "actions, processes, or methodologies that are grounded in and flow from the translation of substantive and current research" (p. 100), where is the evidence to support that the specific activities that faculty engage in while carrying out their teaching roles are "actions, processes, or methodologies that are grounded in and flow from the translation of substantive and current research"? Where is the evidence that directs us in what we should be doing in the role of an academic nurse educator? How do we know if what we are doing is what we should be doing? What competencies define who we are as nurse educators?

Additionally, the National League for Nursing (NLN) supports nurse educators as practicing in a specialty role; that is, teaching in academia requires the knowledge of a specialized practice. In 2005, the NLN issued a position statement titled "Transforming Nursing Education." One of the recommendations in that position statement was, "Faculty identify themselves as advanced practice nurses since teaching is an advanced practice role that requires specialized knowledge and advanced education and since certification now exists as a way to recognize expertise in the role" (NLN, 2005a, p. 5). Finally, there now exists a basis for the evidence for what we do as nurse educators—a certification exam that measures one's knowledge of the "specialized knowledge" of the role of a nurse educator. That is, the answer to the question, "What evidence guides the practice of the academic nurse educator?" is found in the **Certified Nurse Educator (CNE)** examination. The CNE is based on the best practices that define who we are as nurse educators in academia. Evidence now exists for what we are to do in our role as a nurse educator. The value of certification is acknowledged by the NLN because it is viewed as a symbol of professionalism.

This chapter discusses the role of the nurse educator as outlined by the CNE examination and examines the importance of establishing competencies to focus the profession. This chapter provides an overview of the history of the CNE, discusses the test blueprint, gives ideas for preparing for the examination, and concludes with ways the CNE can influence nursing education. The process by which the CNE was conceptualized, studied, and eventually developed is an extraordinary example of an evidence-based activity in nursing education. At this time within nursing education, the CNE certification process is the only course of action available for demonstrating competency for nurse educators. None of the other national organizations and testing entities has developed a certification process system to address the academic nurse educator.

Excellence Through Competencies

To better understand the process involved in the development of a certification process, a clear appreciation of the term **competency** is needed. According to Norman (1985), competency is greater than knowledge alone. It embraces the awareness of knowledge; clinical, technical, and communication skills; and the capacity to decipher a problem through the employing of clinical and/or technical judgment. Competencies are utilized to generate distinctive standards within disciplines and specialties. The clarification of the competencies within a profession allows for the different roles and functions of that position to be effectively and completely addressed and managed by the members of that professional group.

According to Adams and Valiga (2009), "nurses of today and tomorrow need to possess the following qualities: know the principles that underlie their practice; know how to find, manage, and use information; be comfortable with ambiguity and uncertainty; be leaders and change agents; communicate effectively; think critically and from multiple perspectives; function effectively in the face of conflict; and manage constant change, including technological developments"

(p. 2). Just as the competencies of practicing nurses have been studied and delineated, so should the competencies of academic nurse educators. This is evident in the discussion of CNE that is about to unfold in the remainder of this chapter.

The Making of the CNE Examination

Certification in nursing is not a new concept. **Certification** for many nursing specialty practice areas has been available for over 50 years. There is currently a certification for staff development educators provided by the National Nursing Staff Development Organization (NNSDO) and administered by the **American Nurses Credentialing Center (ANCC)**. The exam is the Nursing Professional Development exam. The audience for this examination is strictly nurse educators in healthcare settings, not in academia. Although the role of the staff development educator and the role of the academic nurse educator have much in common, there are also many differences.

A certification exam did not exist that specifically addressed the role of the academic nurse educator. In fact, until recently, the role of the academic nurse educator had not been formally studied and delineated. The NLN provided this valuable information with its research that culminated with the publication of *The Scope of Practice for Academic Nurse Educators* (2005b). This was the first publication that delineated the scope of practice and core competencies of nurse educators.

So, how does an organization such as the NLN go about developing a certification exam for academic nurse educators? Because this is a book about evidence and evidence-based teaching, it would follow that the process used must involve evidence based on research, and that is just what occurred. **Figure 10-1** delineates the steps the NLN followed to establish an evidence-based certification exam.

Think Tank

In 1999, the NLN conducted a Delphi survey that included two questions related to faculty certification. One question asked if the NLN should develop a certification program, and the other asked if members would be interested in seeking certification. The results indicated an extremely positive response to these questions (Ortelli, 2010). With the interest in a certification exam documented, in December 2001, the NLN convened the Think Tank on Graduate Education Preparation for the Nurse Educator Role. The **think tank** was composed of experts in nursing education, who were viewed as master nurse educators, and higher education, with a variety of institutions and backgrounds represented (Halsted, 2007). The think tank was charged

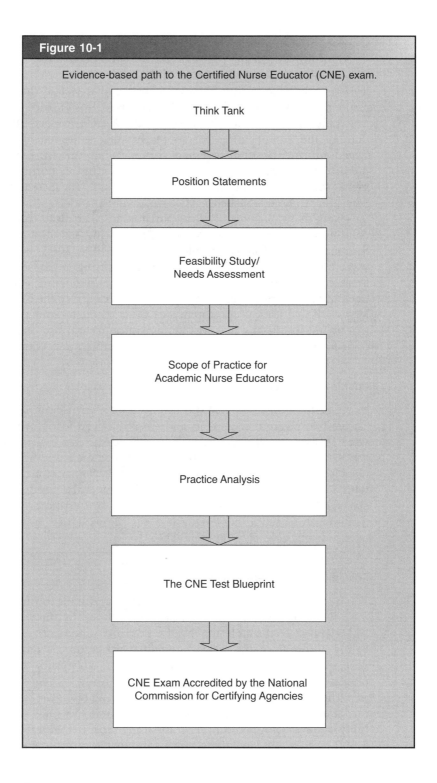

Figure 10-1

Evidence-based path to the Certified Nurse Educator (CNE) exam.

Think Tank

Position Statements

Feasibility Study/
Needs Assessment

Scope of Practice for
Academic Nurse Educators

Practice Analysis

The CNE Test Blueprint

CNE Exam Accredited by the National
Commission for Certifying Agencies

to answer the question: What do educators need to know, or be able to do, to implement the role successfully and effectively?

To reflect a complete picture of the academic nurse educator, all levels of academic institutions were considered as well as the various responsibilities of all levels of the educator role, from novice educator to expert educator. From this data, the think tank produced the first draft of the competencies for academic nurse educators. The NLN issued a formal position statement, summarizing this work, when it published *The Preparation of Nurse Educators* (2002). In this position statement, the NLN specifically recommended that "competence as an educator can be established, recognized, and expanded through master's and/or doctoral education, post-master's certificate programs, continuing professional development, mentoring activities and professional certification as a faculty member" (NLN, 2002, p. 3). This was a bold step for the NLN to take because starting in the late 1980s, most colleges and universities ceased to offer a nursing education track in their graduate nursing programs. This call from the NLN challenged the education community to offer graduate-level programs that would specifically prepare nursing educators and also opened the door for professional certification as an academic nurse educator.

Position Statements

In the early 2000s, the NLN was calling for a reform in nursing education. Two position statements addressed the need for reform. These were *The Preparation of Nurse Educators* (2002) and *Innovation in Nursing Education: A Call to Reform* (2003). Both position statements addressed the need for preparation for the nurse educator role. Preparation as a nurse with a practice specialty is not enough. The nurse also needs the specialized knowledge and skills of the educator. Certification would demonstrate that the nurse educator has the expertise necessary to engage in the role of an academician.

Feasibility Study/Needs Assessment

The need for faculty to attain the knowledge and skills to function in the role of the academician had been established by the think tank and elaborated through the NLN's position statements. However, before committing the human and financial resources required to develop a certification exam, it was necessary to ensure the target population of academic nurse educators was ready.

The NLN assembled various committees and task groups to study this issue. To start, the NLN administered a survey to study the feasibility of developing a certification for academic nurse educators. Over 3,000 respondents, including nurse administrators and nurse faculty, answered the electronic survey. The results indicated that 84% of deans and directors recognized the role of a nurse educator as a specialty and 80% believed certification would be beneficial to their nursing programs (Ortelli, 2010). Faculty respondents indicated an even higher percentage, with 92% considering the role of nurse educator as a specialty. Seventy-six percent of the faculty responding indicated an interest in becoming certified (Ortelli, 2010). The results of these surveys provided evidence of the need to pursue the idea of developing a certification exam for academic nurse educators. The **feasibility study** and **needs assessment** revealed a need for a certification exam for academic nurse educators. The NLN was ready to take the next steps.

Scope of Practice for Academic Nurse Educator: Nurse Educator Competencies

The work of the task group and the findings from the feasibility study set the stage for the NLN to continue its efforts that eventually resulted in the CNE examination. The question to be considered at this point was, "What is the **scope of practice** of an academic nurse educator?" That is, what activities, roles, and knowledge define what the educator does, or **nurse educator competencies**? The answer to this question would require an intense search of the literature to reveal research that provided evidence about the scope of practice of the academic nurse educator. The members of NLN's Task Group on Nurse Educator Competencies searched the literature published between 1992 and 2004 and produced an evidence-based report that characterized the knowledge, skills, and attitudes required of academic nurse educators. However, the report appeared to lack some important competencies the task group members knew were part of the educator's role. Therefore, the task group turned to nonresearch literature to derive a more complete picture of the scope of practice by drawing upon best practices and exemplars to complete the picture (Halstead, 2007). The task group then developed the initial draft of the core competencies with task statements that provided a comprehensive look at the scope of practice of academic nurse educators (NLN, 2005b). These competencies were subsequently reviewed, revised, and refined after perusal and feedback from nurse educators across the country. The initial competencies were:

- Facilitate learning
- Facilitate learner development and socialization
- Use assessment and evaluation strategies
- Participate in curriculum design and evaluation of program outcomes

▓ Function as a change agent and leader
▓ Pursue continuous quality improvement in the nurse educator role
▓ Engage in scholarship
▓ Function within the educational environment

The first draft of the core competencies represented the results of a tremendous evidence-based undertaking by the NLN task group. Within each of these areas delineated by the core competencies, specific standards and hallmarks were organized from the evidence.

These master nursing educators continued the presentation of their work by publishing *Nurse Educator Competencies: Creating an Evidence-Based Practice for Nurse Educators* (Halstead, 2007). This publication provides an explanation of the evidence used to develop the nurse educator competencies. The book presents a synthesis of the research, the gaps in research identified by the task group, and proposed questions that can be used by educators for future research on the many aspects of the role of the nurse academician.

Practice Analysis

The work of the NLN task group that produced the nurse educator competencies and task statements provided a foundation for the CNE **practice analysis**. To ensure the validity of an exam that provides certification or licensure, a practice analysis is used to reveal the activities of the professional engaged in that practice. That is, a practice analysis reveals the activities the professional undertakes while carrying out the roles and responsibilities within the scope of practice of that professional role. The certification exam then tests the candidate's knowledge of those activities.

The NLN assembled a Practice Analysis Committee (PAC) that consisted of eight nurse educators representing faculty in academic settings from diverse geographic, ethnic, and nursing education program types (Ortelli, 2010). Their tasks included:

▓ Developing a sampling plan
▓ Identifying tasks for a survey instrument
▓ Classifying core tasks
▓ Developing a rating scale with demographic variables relevant to those who might take the examination

A survey tool was developed to gather information about the tasks engaged in by academic nurse educators. To develop the survey tool, the committee members used the previously developed core competencies of nurse educators (NLN, 2005b) and examined position descriptions from a number of academic institutions. The resulting survey consisted of 25 demographic variables and a list of job responsibilities or task statements. Those surveyed were to rate the significance of each task statement using a six-point Likert-type scale ranging from "not part of my job" to "of maximum significance."

The practice analysis survey was administered to randomly selected academic nurse educators in all levels of nursing education (Ortelli, 2006). The resultant information gleaned from the survey was judged as adequately or completely addressing the responsibilities of the academic nurse educator. As a result of this practice analysis survey, the CNE exam addresses academic nurse educators who are teaching at any level—LPN, ADN, BSN, and graduate. The examination addresses the role of the academic nurse educator, not any specific educational level.

The CNE Test Blueprint

A final list of 119 tasks was developed and used as the basis for the detailed **test blueprint** that guides the composition of the questions on the CNE. Major categories for the CNE test blueprint developed by the PAC are similar to the major areas of the original nurse educator competencies, with a slight change in verbiage and some of the competencies becoming subconcepts. That is, "Function Within the Educational Environment" became "Engage in Scholarship, Service, and Leadership." "Function as a Change Agent and Leader" and "Engage in Scholarship of Teaching" became subcompetencies under "Engage in Scholarship, Service, and Leadership." **Figure 10-2** aligns the core competencies as established by the task force with the major competencies and hallmarks of the CNE exam.

The final step in developing the test plan was to weight each of the content areas according to significance of the task and breadth of the content within each major area (Ortelli, 2010). Areas of content with higher significance ratings were assigned a greater number of questions. After considering the item distribution that spans the major and minor content areas, the PAC members agreed that 130 items would be sufficient to obtain an acceptable sampling of content to ensure the exam is reliable. The total number of items on the exam is currently 150 items, with 20 items not scored that are being tested for future use. The PAC members elected to restrict the cognitive levels for the test items to three different levels—recall, application, and analysis. The test items are provided as four-option, multiple-choice questions. At this time, test questions are developed by individuals who have successfully completed the CNE examination. Each suggested test question is carefully and thoroughly reviewed to ensure that it meets and addresses a major content area while also meeting an appropriate cognitive level.

Figure 10-2	
Core competences and major content areas.	
Core Competencies	**Major Content Areas of the CNE Exam**
Competency I: Facilitate Learning	Category 1: Facilitate Learning
Competency II: Facilitate Learner Development and Socialization	Category 2: Facilitate Learner Development and Socialization
Competency III: Use Assessment and Evaluation Strategies	Category 3: Use Assessment and Evaluation Strategies
Competency IV: Participate in Curriculum Design and Evaluation of Program Outcomes	Category 4: Participate in Curriculum Design and Evaluation of Program Outcomes
Competency V: Function as a Change Agent and Leader	Category 5: Pursue Continuous Quality Improvement in the Academic Nurse Educator Role
Competency VI: Pursue Continuous Quality Improvement in the Nurse Educator Role	Category 6: Engage in Scholarship, Service, and Leadership
	Subcategory 6A: Function as a Change Agent and Leader
	Subcategory 6B: Engage in Scholarship of Teaching
	Subcategory 6C: Function Effectively Within the Institutional Environments and the Academic Community

Source: National League for Nursing. (2009). *Certified Nurse Educator (CNE) 2010 candidate handbook.* Carbondale, IL: National League for Nursing Academic Nurse Educator Certification Program. Used with permission.

The test blueprint was then completed and determined to represent current practice activities of a full-time academic nurse educator in the United States. It is important to note that the practice analysis targeted the role of the full-time nurse educator. That is, it is only valid and reliable as a certification for those employed full-time. The roles and responsibilities of part-time or adjunct faculty are quite different; therefore, a separate practice analysis and test blueprint would be required for certification of part-time faculty. **Figure 10-3** presents the major content areas and percent of questions for each area.

CNE Exam Accredited by the National Commission for Certifying Agencies (NCCA)

A mark of excellence for nursing programs is accreditation by an outside organization, such as the National League for Nursing Accrediting

Figure 10-3

CNE test blueprint.

Major Content Areas	Percent of Examination
1. Facilitate Learning	25%
2. Facilitate Learner Development and Socialization	11%
3. Use Assessment and Evaluation Strategies	15%
4. Participate in Curriculum Design and Evaluation of Program Outcomes	19%
5. Pursue Continuous Quality Improvement in the Academic Nurse Educator Role	12%
6. Engage in Scholarship, Service, and Leadership	
6A. Function as a Change Agent and Leader	8%
6B. Engage in Scholarship of Teaching	5%
6C. Function Effectively within the Institutional Environment and the Academic Community	5%

Source: National League for Nursing. (2009). *Certified Nurse Educator (CNE) 2010 candidate handbook.* Carbondale, IL: National League for Nursing Academic Nurse Educator Certification Program. Used with permission.

Commission or the Commission on Collegiate Nursing Education. The **National Commission for Certifying Agencies (NCCA)** has a parallel accreditation that indicates excellence. The NCCA evaluates certifying agencies using its established *NCCA Standards for the Accreditation of Certification Programs.* The NLN's CNE Commission was granted accreditation for the CNE Program on April 1, 2009. This was the final step in ensuring the CNE exam is evidence-based because the evidence documented by the NLN while establishing the CNE exam was further confirmed by an accreditation organization outside the NLN. This accreditation also ensures that certification programs adhere to the standards of practice of the certification industry. Therefore, the CNE exam is legitimatized both internally by the NLN and externally by the NCCA.

Eligibility for Taking the CNE Exam

Faculty desiring to take the CNE exam must meet specific criteria. All faculty members must hold an active RN license. The educational requirement is to hold a master's or doctoral degree in nursing. The graduate degree should have a major emphasis in nursing education; if not, the course of study should have provided nine or more credit hours of graduate-level education courses, excluding research or statistics.

Within the NLN CNE *Candidate Handbook* (2009), the mission for the Academic Nurse Educator Certification Program is designated as recognizing "excellence in the advanced specialty role of the academic nurse educator" (p. 2). The goals for the CNE certification are designated as:

- Distinguish academic nursing education as a specialty area of practice and an advanced practice role within professional nursing.
- Recognize the academic nurse educator's specialized knowledge, skills, and abilities and excellence in practice.
- Strengthen the use of core competencies of nurse educator practice.
- Demonstrate a commitment to professional development, lifelong learning, and nursing education as a career. (NLN, 2009, p. 2)

The concepts and expectations suggested by these goals hold the participants to a high level of quality and excellence. The certification is designed to address academic nurse educators from diverse settings. The process is established to allow faculty members to be successful without regard to the manner of educational delivery—traditional classroom-based environments and/or nontraditional environments (e.g., distance delivery via video, closed circuit television, and the Internet). The certification designation is valid for a 5-year period. The NLN has developed a certification renewal process, which reflects that the CNE has continued to demonstrate quality improvement in the academic nurse educator role.

Eligibility for taking the CNE exam includes experience as a full-time nursing educator. *Full-time* is defined by the institution in which the faculty member is employed. For faculty with a master's or doctoral degree in nursing with a major emphasis in nursing education, the experience requirement is 2 years. For those faculty with a master's or doctoral degree in nursing with a major emphasis on a role other than nursing education, the experience requirement is 4 years of full-time employment in the academic faculty role. This is in contrast with the eligibility requirement for other advanced nursing practices, which typically do not require experience—the candidate is eligible to take the certification exam immediately upon completion of graduate nursing education. There are several reasons for the difference. First, for those advanced nursing practices that are regulated by boards of nursing, the nurse practice acts often require the graduate to hold certification as a requirement for the advanced practice license. Second, most advanced practice graduate programs require hundreds of hours of clinical experience in the graduate program. Most masters in nursing education programs require less than 100 hours in a practice practicum. Therefore, graduates from a master's or doctoral-level nursing education program do not have the experience required to pass the certification exam. Time spent working in a full-time faculty position helps the candidate hone the necessary skills.

Preparing to Take the CNE Exam

As with all national exams, it behooves the candidate to prepare for the CNE. There are a number of resources available for this preparation. The CNE *Candidate Handbook* can be accessed from the NLN's website. This handbook provides extensive information about the examination and the procedure for taking the exam. A detailed test plan is included, which is invaluable as a guide for study. The handbook also contains explanations about the testing center, the procedures implemented at the testing center, and a sample screen shot of the test as taken on the computer. Also included is a list of suggested reading materials.

The handbook contains sample questions with their cognitive level. Most of the questions are written at the recall, application, or analysis cognitive levels. However, for a more intense practice experience, the NLN offers an online practice exam called the Self-Assessment Exam (SAE). There are 65 items on the practice exam, which covers all areas of the test blueprint in the same distribution as those of the actual exam. Taking this exam provides the candidate with a tool that diagnoses areas of strength and those that need to be studied to be successful on the actual exam. It also provides the candidate with experience in answering CNE-type questions. The candidate can view rationales for correct and incorrect answers.

The CNE examination has gained popularity over the last 5 years and is perceived as a mark of excellence for both the individual faculty and the nursing program in which the CNE is employed. Therefore, many schools are encouraging their entire faculty to take the CNE exam. In these cases, preparation can be a group affair. One approach to a group study plan includes the following steps:

■ Obtain all the books on the recommended reading list and any other publications that faculty members believe can be helpful.
■ Provide an on-site review session for the entire faculty.

■ Schedule weekly meetings, such as a 2- to 3-hour time block on a specific day, when all faculty members can meet for study sessions.

■ Each week one of the major areas of the CNE test blueprint is presented by assigned faculty followed by discussion of application of the content to practice.

As the faculty group develops strategies for addressing the different aspects covered within the examination, an individualized program of study can be developed. One key aspect when developing a group study plan is the commitment to the study process and the clarification of the time table. Each member of the group must accept and pledge to participate as the different aspects are managed.

As the process for successfully managing the academic nurse educator certification has moved forward, several knowledgeable individuals and groups have developed and offered workshops to help individuals prepare for the examination. Each of these workshops is unique and based upon the individual and/or group presenting the activity.

Application of the content to one's own practice is an extremely valuable exercise that assists the individual faculty to work in-depth with the content, providing meaningful learning. It also provides evidence that the faculty member is indeed engaging in the activities of the nurse academician. This exercise raises one's awareness of one's role. A tool that is helpful with this exercise is found in **Table 10-1**. This tool can also be used for faculty when planning their personal or professional development activities and to document how they are carrying out their role as a nurse academician.

Impact of the CNE on Nursing Education

Holding the CNE credential is a mark of excellence. Those who have passed the CNE are viewed as leaders in nursing education. Those holding the CNE are called upon to contribute to the science of nursing education and to serve as role models in moving forward the specialty area of nursing education.

Additionally, the core competencies that serve as the basis for the CNE test blueprint delineate the activities of the academic nurse educator. Therefore, these provide the basis for developing the curricula of MSN programs in nursing education, thus providing an evidence base for those programs. Currently, there is not a common core of knowledge from nursing education research that is evident in all of these programs. Many programs are based on general education practice. General education is important as core content; however, general

Table 10-1

Faculty Development Tool Related to the Roles of the Academic Nurse Educator

Competencies of the Academic Nurse Educator (Ortelli, 2010)	Examples of How This Competency Is Used in My Teaching	Identified Areas for Faculty Development	Source of Study and Projected Date of Study for Identified Areas for Development
Facilitate Learning			
Facilitate Learner Development and Socialization			
Use Assessment and Evaluation Strategies			
Participate in Curriculum Design and Evaluation of Program Outcomes			
Pursue Continuous Quality Improvement in the Academic Nurse Educator Role			
Engage in Scholarship, Service, and Leadership			
Function as a Change Agent and Leader			
Engage in Scholarship of Teaching			
Function Effectively Within the Institutional Environments and the Academic Community			

Source: © 2009, Linda Caputi, Inc. Used with permission.

education practice should provide a foundation that is then applied to nursing education. The following are some examples:

- As learning theories are discussed, those learning theories should be immediately applied to nursing students.
- Nursing students, as an aggregate, often have very specific characteristics that are different from those of the traditional college student.
- Students in graduate-level nursing education programs must learn to apply general education theory to their student population.

Ensuring that the core competencies of the academic nurse educator as operationalized in the CNE test blueprint are spiraled through graduate-level nursing education programs provides an evidence-based structure for those curricula.

NLN Certification Commission

As the NLN moves forward to ensure that the CNE process maintains a high level of quality, the Certification Commission has been established. The Certification Commission is composed of at least five qualified, voting commissioners elected by the NLN membership and NLN Certification Program certificants in good standing. The NLN president appoints three qualified, voting commissioners, with the approval of the NLN Board of Governors. The Commission appoints one voting public commissioner. The NLN bylaws establish that all voting commissioners, except the public commissioner, shall be RNs credentialed as Certified Nurse Educators and in good standing with their state boards of nursing. In addition, the Commission shall be comprised of the following *ex-officio*, nonvoting members: a current member of the Board of Governors, the certification manager, and other qualified persons appointed by the Commission. The Commission is given the direction to facilitate the ongoing certification of this program. It has been charged with the responsibility to assure that the CNE examination maintains accreditation by the National Commission for Certifying Agencies.

Summary Thoughts

When evidence is used to validate the work done by academic nurse educators, the resulting documents are strong and effectively positioned to address the changing work of nursing education. Each and every step within the process of establishing and maintaining a certification examination to showcase the uniqueness of the specialty of nursing education is strengthened and championed by the work done by the NLN. This group of individuals realized the importance of engaging in the discussion concerning the distinctiveness of the role of the academic nurse educator. As a result of progressing in a logical and organized manner from utilizing experts to thinking about the role, developing positions statements to denote the individuality of the role, engaging in feasibility study and needs assessment activities, establishing a scope of practice, to finally conducting a practice analysis that resulted in a test blueprint, the end product provides a complete and comprehensive look at the role of the nurse educator.

Summary Points

1. The National Council of State Boards of Nursing's recommendations for evidence-based nursing education for regulation include teaching methods, assimilation of the students into the role of nursing, promoting faculty–student relationships, and other areas of teaching.

2. The National League for Nursing (NLN) supports nurse educators as practicing in a specialty role; that is, teaching in academia requires the knowledge of a specialized practice.

3. *The Scope of Practice for Academic Nurse Educators* (2005b) was the first publication that delineated the scope of practice and core competencies of nurse educators.

4. To reflect a complete picture of the academic nurse educator, all levels of academic institutions were considered as well as the various responsibilities of all levels of the educator role, from novice educator to expert educator.

5. The need for faculty to attain the knowledge and skills to function in the role of the academician had been established by the think tank and elaborated through the NLN's position statements.

6. The initial competencies were: facilitate learning, facilitate learner development and socialization, use assessment and evaluation strategies, participate in curriculum design and evaluation of program outcomes, function as a change agent and leader, pursue continuous quality improvement in the nurse educator role, engage in scholarship, and function within the educational environment.

7. A final list of 119 tasks was developed and used as the basis for the detailed test blueprint that guides the composition of the questions on the CNE.

8. The total number of items on the exam is currently 150 items, with 20 items not scored that are being tested for future use.

9. The PAC members elected to restrict the cognitive levels for the test items to three different levels—recall, application, and analysis.

10. The test items are provided as four-option, multiple-choice questions. At this time, test questions are developed by CNE individuals.

11. Each suggested test question is carefully and thoroughly reviewed to ensure that it meets and addresses a major content area while also meeting an appropriate cognitive level.

12. The NLN's CNE Commission was granted accreditation for the CNE Program on April 1, 2009. This was the final step in assuring the CNE exam is evidence-based, because the evidence documented by the NLN while establishing the CNE exam was further confirmed by an accreditation organization outside the NLN.

13. The CNE exam is legitimatized both internally by the NLN and externally by the NCCA.

14. Faculty desiring to take the CNE must meet specific criteria.

15. The NLN has developed a certification renewal process, which reflects that the CNE has continued to demonstrate quality improvement in the academic nurse educator role.

16. The CNE *Candidate Handbook* can be accessed from the NLN's website. This handbook provides extensive information about the examination and the procedure for taking the exam. A detailed test plan is included, which is invaluable as a guide for study.

17. The NLN offers an online practice exam called the Self-Assessment Exam (SAE). There are 65 items on the practice exam, which covers all areas of the test blueprint in the same distribution as those of the actual exam. Taking this exam provides the candidate with a tool that diagnoses areas of strength and those that need to be studied to be successful on the actual exam.

18. As the NLN moves forward to assure the CNE process maintains a high level of quality, the Certification Commission has been established.

19. The Commission is given the direction to facilitate the ongoing certification of this program. It has been charged with the responsibility to ensure that the CNE examination maintains accreditation by the National Commission for Certifying Agencies.

Tips for Nurse Educators

1. Taking the Self-Assessment Exam provides the candidate with a tool that diagnoses areas of strength and those that need to be studied to be successful on the actual exam. It also provides the candidate with experience in answering CNE-type questions. The candidate can view rationales for correct and incorrect answers.

2. For group study in preparation for the exam:
   - Obtain all of the books on the recommended reading list and any other publications that faculty members believe can be helpful.
   - Provide an on-site review session for the entire faculty.
   - Schedule weekly meetings, such as a 2- to 3-hour time block on a specific day, when all faculty members can meet for study sessions.
   - Each week one of the major areas of the CNE test blueprint should be presented by assigned faculty, followed by discussion of application of the content to practice.
   - Each member of the group must accept and pledge to participate as the different aspects are managed.

3. Knowledgeable individuals and groups have developed and offered workshops to help individuals prepare for the examination.

References

Adams, M. H. & Valiga, T. M. (2009). *Achieving excellence in nursing education.* New York, NY: National League for Nursing.

Halstead, J. A. (Ed.). (2007), *Nurse educator competencies: Creating an evidence-based practice for nurse educators.* New York, NY: National League for Nursing.

National League for Nursing. (2002). *Position statement: The preparation of nurse educators.* New York, NY: Author.

National League for Nursing. (2003). *Position statement: Innovation in nursing education: A call to reform.* New York, NY: Author.

National League for Nursing. (2005a). *Position statement: Innovation in nursing education: Transforming nursing education.* New York, NY: Author.

National League for Nursing. (2005b). *The scope of practice for academic nurse educators.* New York, NY: Author.

National League for Nursing. (2009). *Certified Nurse Educator (CNE) 2010 candidate handbook.* Carbondale, IL: National League for Nursing Academic Nurse Educator Certification Program.

National League for Nursing Accrediting Commission. (2008). *NLNAC accreditation manual.* Atlanta, GA: Author.

Norman, G. (1985). *Assessing clinical competence.* New York, NY: Springer.

Ortelli, T. (2006). Defining the professional responsibilities of academic nurse educators: The results of a national practice analysis. *Nursing Education Perspectives, 27*(5), 242–246.

Ortelli, T. (2010). The Certified Nurse Educator credential. In L. Caputi (Ed.), *Teaching nursing: The art and science* (pp. 564–585). Glen Ellyn, IL: College of DuPage Press.

Spector, N. (2006). *Systematic review of students of nursing education outcomes: An evolving review.* Chicago, IL: National Council of State Boards of Nursing.

Web Links

The National Council of State Boards of Nursing (NCSBN) home page is available at www.ncsbn.org.

The National League for Nursing Accrediting Commission (NLNAC) home page is available at www.nlnac.org/home.htm.

Information about the Certified Nurse Educator (CNE) credential is available at www.nln.org/facultycertification/index.htm.

View the American Nurses Credentialing Center (ANCC) home page at www.nursecredentialing.org.

The National Commission for Certifying Agencies (NCCA) home page is available at www.credentialingexcellence.org.

Information about the NLN's Hallmarks of Excellence in Nursing Education is available at www.nln.org/excellence/hallmarks_indicators.htm.

Multiple Choice Questions

1. Which organization offers the CNE examination?

A. AACN
B. ANCC
C. NCSBN
D. NLN

Rationale:

A certification exam did not exist that specifically addressed the role of the academic nurse educator. In fact, until recently, the role of the academic nurse educator had not been formally studied and delineated. The NLN recognized the need and developed the CNE examination.

2. What is the purpose of a task analysis?

A. Provide validly for the content of an exam
B. Determine the feasibility of offering an exam
C. Determine if there is a market for a specific exam
D. Decide who the target audience of an exam will be

Rationale:

To ensure validity of an exam that provides certification or licensure, a practice analysis is used to reveal the activities of the professional engaged in that practice. That is, a practice analysis reveals the activities the professional undertakes while carrying out the roles and responsibilities within the scope of practice of that professional role. The certification exam then tests the candidate's knowledge of those activities.

3. Which statement describes a reason for the need for a certification exam for academic nursing faculty?

A. Teaching nursing is a specialty area.
B. Faculty will earn a higher salary if they are certified.
C. Nursing accrediting bodies require faculty to be certified.
D. Graduates of MSN programs require their students to pass the exam.

Rationale:

Preparation as a nurse with a practice specialty is not enough. The nurse also needs the specialized knowledge and skills of the educator. Certification would demonstrate that the nurse educator has the expertise necessary to engage in the role of an academician.

4. The CNE exam is written for academic nurse educators teaching at which level?

A. LPN
B. ADN
C. BSN and graduate
D. All levels

Rationale:

As a result of the practice analysis survey, the CNE exam addresses academic nurse educators who are teaching at any level—LPN, ADN, BSN, and graduate. The examination addresses the role of the academic nurse educator, not any specific educational level.

5. Which is the primary reason for conducting a feasibility study prior to developing the CNE exam?

   A. Ensure the cost of development can be recovered
   B. Confirm the target population is ready for such an exam
   C. Determine a fair market price for the exam
   D. Ensure schools will reimburse faculty for the cost of the exam

Rationale:

The feasibility study revealed a need for a certification exam for academic nurse educators. NLN was ready to take the next steps.

6. During the development of the CNE exam, a practice analysis survey was administered. To whom was this survey administered?

   A. Nursing program administrators
   B. Nursing students
   C. Developers of graduate-level programs in nursing education
   D. Academic nurse educators

Rationale:

The practice analysis survey was administered to randomly selected academic nurse educators in all levels of nursing education (Ortelli, 2006). The resultant information gleaned from the survey was judged as adequately or completely addressing the responsibilities of the academic nurse educator.

7. How many questions compose the CNE exam?

   A. 75
   B. 100
   C. 130
   D. 150

Rationale:

The total number of items on the exam is currently 150 items, with 20 items not scored that are being tested for future use. The PAC members elected to restrict the cognitive levels for the test items to three different levels—recall, application, and analysis. The test items are provided as four-option, multiple-choice questions. At this time, test questions are developed by CNE individuals. Each suggested test question is carefully and thoroughly reviewed to ensure that it meets and addresses a major content area while also meeting an appropriate cognitive level.

8. What is the minimum number of years of experience required for graduates of an MSN in nursing education to render the candidate eligible to take the CNE exam?

  A. 1
  B. 2
  C. 4
  D. 5

Rationale:

Eligibility for taking the CNE exam includes experience as a full-time nursing educator. Full-time is defined by the institution in which the faculty member is employed. For faculty with a master's or doctoral degree in nursing with a major emphasis in nursing education, the experience requirement is 2 years. For those faculty with a master's or doctoral degree in nursing with a major emphasis on a role other than nursing education, the experience requirement is 4 years of full-time employment in the academic faculty role.

9. Which content area is assigned the largest percent of questions on the CNE exam?

  A. Facilitate learning
  B. Use assessment and evaluation strategies
  C. Participate in curriculum design and evaluation of program outcomes
  D. The combined subcategories included under Engage in Scholarship, Service, and Leadership

Rationale:

See Figure 10-3. The major content area of facilitating learning accounts for 25% of the total questions provided.

10. What is the expectation for those who hold the CNE credential?

  A. Serve as leaders in nursing education
  B. Contribute to the science of nursing education
  C. Serve as a role model in moving forward the specialty area of nursing education
  D. All of the above

Rationale:

See Figure 10-2. As one looks at the core competencies and major content areas, each of the components is evident in the material included within the role of the academic nurse educator.

11. The NLN Certification Commission is composed of

  A. five qualified voting commissioners.
  B. three qualified voting commissioners.
  C. no nonvoting members.
  D. two voting public commissioners.

Rationale:

The Commission is composed of at least five qualified, voting commissioners elected by the NLN membership and NLN Certification Program certificants in good standing. The NLN president appoints three qualified, voting commissioners, with the approval of the NLN Board of Governors. The Commission appoints one voting public commissioner. In addition, the Commission shall be comprised of the following *ex-officio*, nonvoting members: a current member of the Board of Governors, the certification manager, and other qualified persons appointed by the Commission.

12. All members serving on the NLN Certification Commission except the public commissioner must:

A. be members of the NLN.
B. be credentialed as a Certified Nurse Educator.
C. hold a certification of some type.
D. be a member of the NLN Board of Governors.

Rationale:

The bylaws for NLN establish that all voting commissioners, except the public commissioner, shall be RNs credentialed as Certified Nurse Educators and in good standing.

Discussion Questions

1. The entire faculty in one nursing program would like to take the CNE exam. What kinds of activities might help prepare the faculty?

Considerations:

- Form study groups and plan set days/times to work through the content.
- Review all the study materials on the reading list in the CNE *Candidate Handbook*.
- Take the online self-assessment examination to identify areas that need to be studied.
- Examine the CNE test blueprint to identify areas that need to be studied.

2. You would like to develop a certification examination for a specific area of practice. How would you go about such a task?

Considerations:

Refer to Figure 10-1 and lay out the tasks similar to what the NLN did to develop the CNE exam.

Chapter 11

Future Perspectives

Carol Boswell and Sharon Cannon

Chapter Objectives

At the conclusion of this chapter, the learner will be able to:

1. Identify the emergence, impact, and connection of evidence-based teaching for current and future directions in nursing education.
2. Discuss the role of the nurse educator in evidence-based teaching.
3. Utilize teaching strategies/techniques in a variety of educational settings.
4. Identify the role of competencies and certification for nurse educators in the current and future nursing education venues.
5. Explore nursing education research.

Key Terms

➤ Coach

➤ Evidence-based teaching

➤ Institute of Medicine

➤ Mentorship

➤ Preceptor

➤ Robert Wood Johnson Foundation

➤ Translational research

Introduction

Nurse educators have often taught as they were taught. According to Benner, Sutphen, Leonard, and Day (2010), "the central goal of nursing education is for the learner to develop an attuned, response-based practice and capacity to quickly recognize the nature of whole situations in terms of most pressing and least pressing concerns" (p. 43). However, the recent emergence of evidence-based practice (EBP) with a focus on utilization of evidence to provide the best outcomes for nursing has prompted nurse educators to seek the best evidence for student learning outcomes. In addition, the nursing shortage has impacted nurse educators as demands for increased enrollments, recruitment, and retention of students require nurse educators to explore strategies and skills to accommodate those demands through unique and innovative approaches that are grounded in solid evidence. Compounding the problem resulting from the nursing shortage is the aging population of both the nursing workforce and nurse educators. Aging of the workforce and nursing faculty resulted in a 2010 joint statement of the Tri-Council for Nursing, in which Dr. Peter Buerhaus indicated, "currently, nearly 900,000 RNs (out of the estimated 2.6 million working RNs) are over the age of 50, and large numbers of these RNs are expected to retire in the years ahead (independent of the pace and intensity of a jobs recovery)" (AACN, 2010a, p. 4). Buerhaus further noted that replacement of the aging RNs and increasing the supply of RNs will be needed. The Tri-Council also suggested that the capacity of nursing education programs must increase. Consequently, nurse educators will be challenged to not only manage larger classes, but also to increase graduation rates and successful passages of the NCLEX examination. The demands on the nurse educator mandate that these areas be considered. As schools work to increase fiscal responsibility, faculty members are confronted with larger classes and more demands to ensure the success rate for the students.

The preceding chapters have been designed to provide a foundation for both novice and experienced faculty to build their knowledge and skills in the nursing education arena on evidence rather than relying on a "gut feeling" or past educational experience. Agencies outside of nursing, such as the **Institute of Medicine** (IOM) and **Robert Wood Johnson Foundation**, have emphasized the need for **evidence-based teaching** (EBT) and nurse educators who have the skills and abilities to teach in nursing education today and in the future to meet the demands for a well-prepared healthcare workforce.

Let's see how the preceding chapters fit for EBT for current and future directions. Fostering the future EBT perspective begins with the development of the role of the academician regarding the provision of preceptors/coaches and mentors, the ethics of teaching, utilization of multiple settings, teaching methodologies in various settings, evaluation, current EBT research, and establishing the competency of the nurse educator.

Preceptor/Coach

According to the American Heritage® Dictionary of the English Language (2009), the definition for **preceptor** is "an expert or specialist, such as a physician, who gives practical experience and training to a student" (p. 1). Preceptors are frequently utilized to support and expand the learning environment for students. The same source provides the definition for **coach** as "a private tutor employed to prepare a student for an examination" (American Heritage® Dictionary of the English Language, 2009, p. 1). Within the nursing field, a coach is a private expert or specialist who works directly with a student to aid the acquisition of knowledge. Clinically competent nurses are called upon in many settings to provide the support and practical experience for students to allow for the advancement of the knowledge base. Didactic teaching settings are established to accentuate the cognitive domain of learning. Clinical instructors, preceptors, and coaches are required to translate the cognitive knowledge to the psychomotor and affective domains through application. From the evidence, Modic and Schoessler (2010) identified fours themes that preceptors identified as key areas needing to be strengthened: "(1) learning how to capitalize on teaching moments, (2) applying evidence-based teaching, (3) providing constructive performance feedback, and (4) adapting teaching strategies to match the different learning needs of students" (p. 134). Each of these areas is paramount as orientation programs for preceptors and coaches are established, and as preceptors/coaches are supported and developed. Individuals who agree to serve as preceptors and coaches for the next generation of students want to support and develop the novice nurses in a positive and encouraging manner. The idea of "eating our young" is not the feedback which most nurses desire. In reality, the strengthening and championing of the next generation of nurses is the ultimate goal for individuals who accept the responsibility of precepting and coaching student nurses.

Manion (2010) wrote that "generational diversity was widely popularized in the early nineties when the advent of large numbers of GenXers into our workforce caused many Baby Boomers to shake their heads in bewilderment" (p. 8). The idea of groups of individuals precepting each other while holding differing values, attitudes, and work goals caused increased anxiety within the workplace. Multiple studies have been done to help validate the differences between the values, interests, and tactics to best use with the different groupings. Manion (2010) notes that little evidence was located related to specific leadership strategies that are effective based upon generational differences alone. In reality, the challenges and rewards confronted within the precepting/coaching experience are based upon the complexity of the workforce resulting from geographical, cultural, ethnic, generational, and professional diversity. No one aspect is the primary driver, but instead the intricacy of each individual as multiple forces come to bear on the development of that individual must be considered. From the research completed by Manion (2010), five basic human intrinsic motivators were identified as contributing to the creation of a dynamic work environment. Preceptors and coaches can utilize these five motivators as they strive to aid the learners toward their educational goals. The five motivators are: healthy relationships (positive, healthy working interactions), meaningful work (perceived by the individual as worthwhile and fulfilling), competence (building on strengths to advance self), autonomy (having authority to make decisions and implement actions), and progress (realizing that activities completed have had an impact).

Mentorship

The American Heritage® Dictionary of the English Language (2009) defines **mentor** as "a wise and trusted counselor or teacher, to serve as a trusted counselor or teacher, especially in occupational settings, and/or to serve as a trusted counselor or teacher to (another person)" (p. 1). The concept of mentor differs from the role of preceptor/coach. A mentor is considered to be a long-term commitment to the development of an individual. Preceptors and coaches are selected and appointed for a specific time period or grouping of objectives. Mentors are usually mutually selected by the individuals involved instead of being appointed. Within the mentoring process utilized by Latimer and Kimbell (2010), the recommendation was made to allow the mentoring process to have one-on-one consultation time rather than requiring mentoring activities to be done as a group action. The relationship established within a mentorship can be viewed as either a protégée/mentor or fellow/mentor. Within each of these relationships, the custom is a one-on-one process directed toward one primary goal. The protégée/mentor or fellow/mentor can identify further goals as the relationship develops, but initially they are connected by a single ambition. As the rapport develops, further aspects may be ascertained that will allow the relationship to mature in a different way.

Barnsteiner, Reeder, Palma, Preston, and Walton (2010) discuss the use of a mentor program to promote EBP and **translational research**. Within this project, five clinical educators accepted the task of serving as mentors for staff nurses related to EBP and translational research. Over the course of a 1-year fellowship period, these mentors provided support and instruction to the fellows as they moved from novice researchers toward a firmer understanding of the interconnectiveness of EBP and translational research. The mentors served as EBP champions and resource individuals as the designated fellow initiated a project. According to Barnsteiner et al. (2010), the goal was "to fuel a love of knowledge, enthusiasm for questioning the status quo, and interest in exploring new approaches to practice based on emerging science and national standards" (p. 225). Within the mentor process, the love of learning was supported and encouraged.

Another example of the use of mentorship to transform an organizational EBP culture is presented by Ogiehor-Enoma, Taqueban, and Anosike (2010), who note, "a commitment to EBP begins with establishing a culture in which nurses are mentored in developing skills for defining problems and improving clinical decision making in their work environment" (p. 14). Within this example, six steps were used: (1) conducting an organizational inventory, (2) constructing a strong infrastructure for EBP, (3) valuing the EBP process while embracing the different parts, (4) augmenting internal resources via educational venues, (5) embedding the aspects into day-to-day practice, and (6) sustaining the culture change. Ogiehor-Enoma et al. (2010) note the expectation that direct care nurses should acquire an internal consultant, mentors, and coaches to facilitate the complex EBP activities. The use of consultants, mentors, and coaches was viewed as an integral aspect of the success of the transformation. Utilizing the expertise of champions to support and advance the other staff was viewed as a major strength within this process. The culture developed into one of support and encouragement, not competition.

Since mentoring is viewed as longer term than precepting/ coaching, career mapping programs can be an EBT model for the advancement of the protégée/fellow. Shermont, Krepcio, and Murphy (2009) stated that "meeting the demands of complex care environments requires a nursing workforce that is committed to continued learning and to advancing clinical as well as leadership skills" (p. 432). The process of career mapping involves the pairing of a mentor/clinical advisor with an individual to assist the individual to define distinct professional aspirations, cultivate a plan for achieving those goals, and collaborate as the plan is implemented. From the evidence, career planning has been found to empower individuals to chart their own professional path and take responsibility for that journey. Through the use of the mentor/clinical advisor to validate the individual's attempts to chart his or her own course, a sense of confidence can be forthcoming and corroborated. The mentor/clinical advisor can assist the individual to set realistic goals. Once those goals are in place and the individual is committed to strive for them, the mentor/clinical advisor is then used to access resources and act as a cheerleader. This cheerleading/championing of the individual's own plan provides further self-confidence and security. The individual can then develop skills to use in future career growth efforts. The work done by Shermont et al. (2009) resulted in "revitalizing nurses' interest in their careers, the program enhanced nurse satisfaction as well as retention and reduces staff turnover and the attendant nurse replacement costs" (p. 437). By supporting individuals to strive for their own career goals, the agency received the benefit of satisfied employees who were invigorated to strive for quality and recognition. The benefits of this mentoring program resulted in a true "win-win" result for the employer and employee.

Impact of Continued Nursing

Just as nurses at the bedside need to be cognizant of new technologies and the need to keep current on EBP, so too does the nurse educator need to maintain competence and expertise in the realm of being a nurse educator. As efforts to produce more evidence for teaching nursing education occur, faculty will need to continue to add to their knowledge the best practices for obtaining learning outcomes of students and for overall evaluation of themselves, courses, and programs. Institutes for immersion in the faculty role, new technology, workshops/conferences (local, state, and national), postgraduate courses, and journal articles provide a wide array of choices to keep current and up to date on new evidence.

As mentioned previously, the RN workforce is aging. The current projections are that 260,000 new nurses will be needed by 2025 (AACN, 2010b). At the present time approximately 55,000 qualified applications for nursing programs are being turned away (AACN, 2010b). Barriers to increasing enrollments are lack of faculty, clinical sites, and classroom space, as well as economic budgetary restraints. Unfortunately, compounding this issue is the aging of faculty, which will result in even fewer faculty members to teach future programs. However, before predicting doom and gloom, new technology and research in nursing education may offer a ray of hope. Faculty members will be challenged to seek innovative, creative EBT methods to address the pressures that will inevitably be present. Legislative efforts from national and state nursing organizations are working, and will continue to work, to improve the likelihood of increasing under-graduate and graduate funding for nursing education for scholarships, research, new program start-ups, and faculty salaries. In addition, the IOM and the Robert Wood Johnson Foundation conducted three forums across the United States to obtain feedback from recognized leaders in nursing education and clinical agencies to examine the future direction for nursing education. Their report is due to be distributed in the fall of 2010. The Carnegie Foundation for the Advancement of Teaching has also stepped forward though the efforts of Benner et al. (2010), who call for a radical transformation for educating nurses. All of these combined efforts are designed to ensure that the 32 million more citizens of the future will be able to access health care and subsequently nursing care in a variety of settings.

Research in Nursing Education

As was stated in previous chapters, research endeavors within nursing education have ebbed and flowed. At times within our history, federal monies have been available to fund the research projects related to validating educational strategies. At other times, the monies have been scarce. In the current funding environment, some revenue streams are available. Funding sources for nursing education tend to be small grant amounts funded by nursing professional organizations, such as the National League for Nursing (NLN), Sigma Theta Tau International (STTI), and the American Nurses Association (ANA). Federal grant monies continue to be few and far between but primarily can be located within the U.S. Health Resources and Services Administration (HRSA). Projects that combine nursing education and clinical practice seem to be areas where federal monies can be sought. Funding sources for research endeavors related to simulation projects are available through the private sector. Private-sector companies such as Johnson and Johnson and the Robert Wood Johnson Foundation are opening selected funding streams related to specific focal points within each company's strategic plan.

Shortage of Healthcare Workers

Mason (2010) stated that "the new law (Patient Protection and Affordable Care Act—PL111.148) includes federal support for developing the healthcare workforce, including nurses, with a particular emphasis on expanding the number and preparation of primary care providers" (p. 24). Though the media has repeatedly discussed the growing concerns related to the shortages of healthcare workers, this new law adds to the opportunities for change. Improvements in the approaches and tactics to be used as increasing demands are placed on the educational community to meet these demands must be carefully and appropriately considered. Shortages for physician, pharmacists, and nurses, to name a few, will lead to a greater demand. These groups will be called on to accommodate the increased population seeking to access the healthcare services when mandatory health insurance becomes a reality. These demands will stretch the limits for all healthcare practitioners. Each group will be required to provide the resources to address the changes within the healthcare field based upon the federal regulations.

Application to Settings Other Than Academia

Evidence-based teaching will be essential for the preparation of nurses entering the workforce and for continuing competence of nurses. Thus, EBT has a major impact for nurse educators in clinics, hospitals, schools, home health, and hospice agencies. Nursing staff development personnel must also utilize EBT and, just as important, conduct research for the best evidence to teach in areas outside of academia. Keeping abreast of EBT advancements in nursing will assist those nurse educators in the preparation, implementation, and evaluation of programs for nursing staff. Clinical/Career Ladders, Magnet, and Pathway to Excellence status and accreditation agencies such as the Joint Commission will continue to urge education of staff to be a major priority. As a result, nurse educators outside of academia will also use evidence to demonstrate competency outcomes which in turn impact patient outcomes.

Creating a Vision for Evidence-Based Teaching

Senthuran (2010) stated that "the journey to gain understanding and meaning is part of the evolution of nursing as a discipline. It is necessary for a group of people, a culture, to understand what and why they do things to gain a sense of themselves so that they can determine how they fit into the world and how to evolve" (p. 245). As the profession begins to transition toward an EBT affiliation, care should be given to considering a model for the transition from student to competent nursing professional. Faculty members engaged in advancing the success of the educational process must promote the successful transition of students into the actual workplace setting. Another focus for the transition is related to moving novice faculty members toward a confident embracing of the educator role.

Bahouth and Esposito-Herr (2009) embraced the Brown and Olshansky stages for transition from student to competent nurse practitioner. The four stages can be easily incorporated as a means for moving students of any level toward competent healthcare delivery. These same four stages can be applied to advancing the novice faculty member from initial role performance toward a level of secure management of the educational process. The four stages are: (1) laying the foundation, (2) launching, (3) meeting the challenge, and (4) broadening the perspectives. According to Bahouth and Esposito-Herr (2009), the initial period provides the venue for students to move out of the educational process and into the workplace setting. The interlude results in stress for the individuals as they endeavor to determine appropriate work settings. The second stage includes the process of getting involved in the actual work of the job—moving from being that student who is waiting to break into the process to the point of being that individual who assumes a place at the work table with confidence and integrity. The next stage of meeting the challenges allows the individual to build and develop confidence and competence within the work setting selected. The final phase takes place as the student has moved from the learner on the side to a member of the team.

These same four stages can be readily applied to the novice educator. Novice faculty members must be provided the time and resources to lay a firm foundation for the effective management of the learning process. Opportunities for the faculty member to try out these different strategies with diverse student populations are mandatory. The novice faculty member needs to confront the challenges of the diverse student population while having the tools needed to be successful. These individuals should not be thrown out into the raging rapids to sink or swim without having a lifeguard (seasoned faculty member) to help them acquire the different skills and strategies needed to be successful in this different venue of practice. Clinically competent nurses can successfully transition into the educator role but do need to have the opportunities and resources to productively and effectively manage the education environment of the 21st century and beyond.

Within EBT, faculty members need to help the students to understand that this movement from the student role toward a competent member of the team takes time and energy. It is not just that a student acquires pieces of paper (diploma and licenses), and hence the person is ready to take on all aspects of the workplace. Faculty members must acknowledge that it is a process and discover ways to help the student transition toward that exciting new role. Part of understanding EBT is that even within the teaching/education role, evidence is key for helping each member progress toward his or her educational goals.

Benner et al. (2010) strongly suggest four essential shifts needed to actively engage students in a positive manner:

1. Shift from a focus on covering decontextualized knowledge to an emphasis on teaching for a sense of salience, situated cognition, and action in particular situations.
2. Shift from a sharp separation of clinical and classroom teaching to integration of classroom and clinical teaching.
3. Shift from an emphasis on critical thinking to an emphasis on clinical reasoning and multiple ways of thinking that include critical thinking.
4. Shift from an emphasis on socialization and role taking to an emphasis on formation. (pp. 82–86)

With each of these areas, faculty members move from a passive delivery to an active engagement of the students.

Another crucial aspect of utilizing EBT during the transition into practice relates to generational issues. Hudspeth (2009) stated that consideration must be given "to having 4 generations, and sometimes 5, in the same clinical setting at one time" (p. 352). As discussed earlier in this text, the concerns related to harmonizing the work expectations for each of these generations require that faculty carefully consider the needs, attitudes, and expectations for each of the generations. Forethought should be given to how best to engage each of the generations so that a smoother balancing of the opportunities can be ensured. Each of these generations embraces different lifestyles, educational types, and learning styles. Faculty members who are willing to investigate potential approaches for engaging the different groups should meet with a more positive outcome for the learning process. Stereotyping is not appropriate, but realizing the uniqueness of each group can be used to improve the learning process. As faculty members consider the generational issues, attention should be directed to the faculty group makeup, teaching team composition, and committee groups. It is not just about the student population, but all aspects within the teaching environment. Care should be given to understanding our peers, colleagues, and students.

In addition to the generational issues, cultural issues can go hand in hand with this need to welcome the uniqueness and distinctiveness of the different individuals encountered during the learning process. Sherman (2010) entitles this "building generational synergy" (p. 4). Determining a generational profile of the student cohort can aid the instructor to carefully consider the distinct needs that may be present. By establishing this blueprint of the cohort's composition, faculty can use that to build the synergetic environment which allows the group to develop a strong foundation to foster future learning opportunities. While Sherman (2010) acknowledges that the nurse leader is paramount in the environment, the idea can be translated to reflect that the educator holds the strategic position for setting the tone and culture within the learning environment. The faculty member who endeavors to use EBT realizes that the establishment of a culture of inclusion and respect is important and must include generational and cultural beliefs and biases. Sherman (2010) relates that "points of conflict can often be turned into teachable moments" (p. 5). Through the embracing of EBT, faculty members will understand the necessity for utilizing all knowledge to best present and advance the profession of nursing. As areas that can result in "pull back" from positive results are encountered, EBT champions will demand that evidence be sought to ensure that the learning environment is not negatively impacted. An example of this can be seen in the work being done by Gary Small at the University of California Los Angeles (UCLA) (Sherman, 2010). This work is suggesting that the "changes we see in the classroom with students today such as shortened attention spans and skimming of reading material may be a biological adaptation to new technology" (Sherman, 2010, p. 5). Diversity within the learning community allows for the strengths and limitations of each generation to be supported by others within the group. A diverse learning community can better handle the complexity and challenges encountered within the rapidly changing healthcare arena.

Creating a vision of EBT mandates the utilization of technology. The Technology Informatics Guiding Education Reform (TIGER) initiative is an exemplar of EBT. According to Hebda and Calderone (2010), "the 2003 Institute of Medicine report, *Health Professions Education: A Bridge to Quality*, identified 5 core competencies for healthcare professionals: the ability to delivery patient-centered care, the ability to work as members of an interdisciplinary team, the use of evidence-based practice, quality improvement approaches, and informatics" (p. 56). This project embraced the concepts of EBP (thus EBT) to identify the vision/mission/goals, develop informatics competencies, and implement these competencies into nursing education. Through the TIGER initiative, nurse educators have been provided with strategies for integrating technology-enhanced experiences into the lesson plans and curricula. The informatics competencies are divided into all nurses, beginning nurses, and experienced nurses. The evidence has been assembled and harvested from multiple resources to ensure that the TIGER initiative project has the current core competencies that are needed. EBT can and does work to bring together important and needed information to advance the science of nursing and nursing education.

As agencies, groups, and educators begin to carefully and logically consider the idea of EBT, awareness grows that each and every individual has something to offer. Evidence can and does come from many different directions. Nursing must stay vigilant for its individual body of knowledge while embracing knowledge from other disciplines. Krom, Batten, and Bautista (2010) embraced collaboration with a clinical nurse specialist, health science librarian, and staff nurse to advance the EBP process at their institution. Utilizing multiple individuals allowed for an effective collaborative effort that resulted in successful modification of the work environment at an academic medical center. It was found that "each brought an important perspective that would help the staff nurse become familiar with the concept and overcome any personal barrier" (Krom et al., 2010, p. 56). Realizing the expertise that is available through the engagement with other disciplines, departments, and resources opens the opportunities for advancement of the agenda toward EBT and EBP.

Summary Thoughts

According to Ogiehor-Enoma et al. (2010), "in today's era of knowledgeable healthcare consumers, evidence-based practice has become the gold standard as consumers demand quality care that's proven to be effective and safe" (p. 14). If within health care and nursing care, EBP is the gold standard, then can nursing education require anything less than EBT? Just as EBP requires the best evidence, EBT must also accept the challenge to integrate the best-known teaching/educational strategies with clinical expertise and students' values to ensure that the knowledge level is appropriate and of high standards. Senthuran (2010) spoke of the evolution toward the next level. Evidence-based teaching is that process of evolving toward an improved delivery of the art of learning. Ensuring that the different processes used to augment the processes of knowledge acquisition are based upon the best evidence is sensible and logical. As each aspect of EBP and EBT is incorporated into the day-to-day delivery of health care, the outcomes will be improved and validated.

Benner et al. (2010) stated that "high-stakes learning is a necessity; only experiential learning can yield the complex, open-ended, skilled knowledge required for learning to recognize the nature of the particular resources and constraints in equally open-ended and under-determined clinical situations" (p. 42). Nurse educators must accept the challenge to move nursing education toward an evidence-based delivery process which embraces experiential learning. The time for passive learning strategies has passed. Active learning strategies are required in the fast-paced healthcare arena. With the challenges of an aging faculty, nursing shortage, and changing healthcare agendas, the educational process must pull from the evidence to actively engage the students to ensure that they are capable to meet the future challenges to come within nursing and health care.

Valiga (2010) stated that "excellence in teaching involves challenging ourselves and trying to do things beyond what we have already mastered, so that we continue to grow and so that our students' educational experiences are powerful and inspiring" (p. 1). Within EBT, the call and challenge is for each of us as faculty members to strive for the excellence within the educational experience. If we do not reach for the stars and expect the striving for distinction from ourselves and students, where will the nursing profession be in the future? Each of us must embrace the ultimatum to not accept mediocrity, but rather to strive for the highest level within each and every activity that we engage in.

Summary Points

1. The nursing shortage is a result of the aging of the workforce, aging of faculty, and a lack of financial support, clinical sites, and classroom space.
2. Regardless of the clinical setting, continued nursing education of nurse educators is vital for the provision of health care.
3. Research in nursing education has ebbed and flowed but is currently being conducted due to new streams of funding.
4. EBT has a major impact for nurse educators in clinics, hospitals, schools, home health, and hospice agencies.
5. A preceptor is an expert or authority who provides realistic experience and instruction to a student.
6. A coach is an expert or specialist who works with one student directly to help with the dissemination of knowledge.
7. Individuals who agree to serve as preceptors and coaches for the next generation of students want to support and develop the novice nurses in a positive and encouraging manner.
8. The challenges and rewards confronted within the precepting/coaching experience are based upon the complexity of the workforce resulting from geographical, cultural, ethnic, generational, and professional diversity.
9. Five motivators that can be used by preceptors and coaches are healthy relationship, meaningful work, competence, autonomy, and progress.
10. A mentor is considered to hold a long-term commitment to the development of an individual.
11. The process of career mapping involves the pairing of a mentor/clinical advisor with an individual to assist the individual to define distinct professional aspirations, cultivate a plan for achieving those goals, and collaborate as the plan is implemented.
12. Faculty members engaged in advancing the success of the educational process must embrace the idea of promoting the successful transition of students into the actual workforce setting.

13. Part of EBT is understanding that even within the teaching/education role, evidence is key for helping each member progress toward his or her education goals.

14. In addition to the generational issues, cultural issues can go hand in hand with the need to welcome the uniqueness and distinctiveness of the different individuals encountered during the learning process.

15. By establishing a blueprint of the cohort's composition, faculty members can use that to build the synergetic environment that allows the group to develop a strong foundation to foster future learning opportunities.

16. The faculty member who endeavors to use EBT realizes that the establishment of a culture of inclusion and respect is paramount and must include consideration of generational and cultural beliefs and biases.

17. Nursing must stay vigilant for its individual body of knowledge while embracing knowledge from other disciplines.

18. Evidence-based teaching must accept the challenge to integrate the best-known teaching/educational strategies with clinical expertise and students' values to ensure that the knowledge level is appropriate and of high standards.

Tips for Nurse Educators to Use

1. When selecting preceptors and coaches, care should be given to ensure that the individual has the desire to engage with the student to develop the student's knowledge base and skills.

2. Preceptors and coaches strive to impart knowledge and skills for a directed period of time, whereas a mentor works to develop an individual's professional goals over a longer time period.

3. Didactic teaching settings are established to accentuate the cognitive domain of learning.

4. Clinical instructors, preceptors, and coaches are depended upon to translate the cognitive knowledge to the psychomotor and affective domains through application.

5. Continuing nursing education opportunities abound for nurse educators to assist them in their teaching role.

6. EBT activities designed to improve student learning outcomes are essential to add to the body of nursing education knowledge.

7. EBT is not restricted to the academic setting but rather should be actively sought by nursing staff development personnel.

References

American Association of Colleges of Nursing. (2010a). Joint statement from the Tri-Council for Nursing on recent registered nurse supply and demand projections. Retrieved July 28, 2010, from http://www.aacn.nche.edu/Education/pdf/Tricouncilrnsupply.pdf

American Association of Colleges of Nursing. (2010b). Talking points: Impact of the economy on the nursing shortage. Retrieved July 28, 2010, from http://www.aacn.nche.edu/Media/pdf/Economy.pdf

American Heritage® Dictionary of the English Language, 4th ed. (2009). Preceptor. Houghton Mifflin Company. Retrieved July 31, 2010, from http://www.thefreedictionary.com/preceptors

Bahouth, M. N., & Esposito-Herr, M. B. (2009). Orientation program for hospital-based nurse practitioners. *AACN Advanced Critical Care*, 20(1), 82–90.

Barnsteiner, J. H., Reeder, V. C., Palma, W. H., Preston, A. M., & Walton, M. K. (2010). Promoting evidence-based practice and translational research. *Nursing Administrative Quarterly*, 34(3), 217–225.

Benner, P., Sutphen, M., Leonard, V., & Day, L. (2010). *Educating nurses: A call for radical transformation*. San Francisco, CA: Jossey-Bass Higher and Adult Education Series.

Hebda, T., & Calderone, T. L. (2010). What nurse educators need to know about the TIGER initiative. *Nurse Educator*, 35(2), 56–60.

Hudspeth, R. (2009). Regulation's burden regarding transition to practice. *Nursing Administrative Quarterly*, 33(4), 352–354.

Krom, Z. R., Batten, J., & Bautista. C. (2010). A unique collaborative nursing evidence-based practice initiative using the Iowa model: A clinical nurse specialist, a health science librarian, and a staff nurse's success story. *Clinical Nurse Specialist*, 24(2), 54–59.

Latimer, R., & Kimbell, J. (2010). Nursing research fellowship: Building nursing research infrastructure in a hospital. *Journal of Nursing Administration*, 40(2), 92–98.

Manion, J. (2010). The challenges and rewards of an intergenerational workforce. *Voice of Nursing Leadership: The American Organization of Nurse Executives*, 3(4), 8–10.

Mason, D. J. (2010). Health care reform: What's in it for nursing? *American Journal of Nursing*, 110(7), 24–26.

Modic, M. B., & Schoessler, M. (2010). Preceptorship. *Journal for Nurses in Staff Development*, 134–136.

Ogiehor-Enoma, G., Taqueban, L., & Anosike, A., (2010). 6 steps for transforming organizational EBP culture. *Nursing Management*, 14–17.

Senthuran, R. A. (2010). Why ask why? *Nursing Science Quarterly*, 23(3), 245–247.

Sherman, R. (2010). Creating synergy on multigenerational nursing teams. *Voice of Nursing Leadership: The American Organization of Nurse Executives*, 3(4), 4–6.

Shermont, H., Krepcio, D., & Murphy, J. M. (2009). Career mapping: Developing nurse leaders, reinvigorating careers. *Journal of Nursing Administration*, 39(10), 432–437.

Valiga, T. (2010). Excellence: Does the word mean anything anymore? *Journal of Nursing Education*. Guest Editorial.

Web Links

Visit the American Association of Colleges of Nursing at www.aacn.nche.edu.

The National League for Nursing home page is available at www.nln.org.

The American Association of Nursing home page is available at www.nursingworld .org.

The Institute of Medicine home page is available at www.iom.edu.

The Sigma Theta Tau International home page is available at www.nursingsociety.org.

Learn more about the Robert Wood Johnson Foundation at www.rwjf.org.

Visit the Johnson and Johnson home page at www.jnj.com/connect.

Multiple Choice Questions

1. A preceptor is an expert or specialist who provides

    A. practical experience and training for a student.
    B. day-to-day support to a clinical instructor.
    C. one-on-one interaction with a physician.
    D. long-term support to a student.

Rationale:

According to the *American Heritage Dictionary of the English Language* (2009), the definition for preceptor is "an expert or specialist, such as a physician, who gives practical experience and training to a student" (p. 1). Preceptors are frequently utilized to support and expand the learning environment for students.

2. A coach is an expert or specialist who provides

    A. cognitive experience and training for a student.
    B. day-to-day support to a clinical instructor related to affective knowledge.
    C. one-on-one interaction with a student related to practical experience.
    D. long-term support to a student.

Rationale:

The definition for coach is "a private tutor employed to prepare a student for an examination" (*American Heritage Dictionary of the English Language*, 2009, p. 1). Within the nursing field, a coach is a private expert or specialist who does work directly with a student to aid in the acquisition of knowledge.

3. Within the clinical setting, the primary knowledge domains addressed are

    A. cognitive and psychomotor.
    B. psychomotor and affective.
    C. affective and cognitive.
    D. cognitive and psychomotor.

Rationale:

Didactic teaching settings are established to accentuate the cognitive domain of learning. Clinical instructors, preceptors, and coaches are depended upon to translate the cognitive knowledge to the psychomotor and affective domains through application.

4. Modic and Schoessler (2010) identified four themes that preceptors acknowledged as needing to be strengthened to be successful at clinical instruction. One of those themes is to

    A. develop the ability to find the teachable moment.
    B. stick with tried-and-true teaching methods.
    C. utilize negative feedback to make a strong point.
    D. not worry about evidence when trying to make a clinical point.

Rationale:

From the evidence, Modic and Schoessler (2010) identified fours themes that preceptors noted as key areas needing to be strengthened: "(1) learning how to capitalize on teaching moments, (2) applying evidence-based teaching, (3) providing constructive performance feedback, and (4) adapting teaching strategies to match the different learning needs of students" (p. 134). Each of these areas is paramount as orientation programs for preceptors and coaches are established and as preceptors/coaches are supported and developed.

5. Career mapping is a process in which a mentor/clinical advisor and an individual strive to
   A. define organization goals, determine plan for the unit, and implement that plan.
   B. define agency goals, cultivate a plan to achieve those goals, and work to implement it.
   C. define distinct professional aspirations, cultivate a plan for achieving those goals, and collaborate as the plan is implemented.
   D. define distinct personal aspirations, cultivate a plan for achieving agency goals, and collaborate as the plan is implemented.

Rationale:

The process of career mapping involves the pairing of a mentor/clinical advisor with an individual to assist the individual to define distinct professional aspirations, cultivate a plan for achieving those goals, and collaborate as the plan is implemented. From the evidence, career planning has been found to empower individuals to chart their own professional path and take responsibility for that journey.

6. Faculty members who want to build a synergetic environment need to
   A. ignore generational issues, as they are not important.
   B. set the agenda for all classes to reduce stress.
   C. determine the required aspects to ensure that all areas are covered.
   D. set the tone and culture within the learning environment.

Rationale:

Determining a generational profile of the student cohort can aid the instructor to carefully consider the distinct needs which may be present. By establishing this blueprint of the cohort's composition, faculty can use that to build the synergetic environment that allows the group to develop a strong foundation to foster future learning opportunities. While Sherman (2010) acknowledges that the nurse leader is paramount in the environment, the idea can be translated to reflect that the educator holds the strategic position for setting the tone and culture within the learning environment.

7. A key aspect identified by the 2003 Institute of Medicine report is that students need to have developed competencies in

    A. managed care.

    B. generalist skills.

    C. medication administration.

    D. informatics.

Rationale:

This project embraced the concepts of EBP (and thus EBT) to identify the vision/mission/goals, develop informatics competencies, and implement these competencies into nursing education. Through the TIGER initiative, nurse educators have been provided with strategies for integrating technology-enhanced experiences into lesson plans and curricula. The informatics competencies are divided into those for all nurses, beginning nurses, and experienced nurses.

8. The current nursing shortage is most impacted by:

    A. lack of interest in nursing.

    B. aging of the workforce and faculty.

    C. little support from national nursing organizations.

    D. too many other professions from which to choose.

Rationale:

Aging of the workforce and nursing faculty resulted in a 2010 joint statement of the Tri-Council for Nursing, in which Dr. Peter Buerhaus indicated, "currently, nearly 900,000 RNs (out of the estimated 2.6 million working RNs) are over the age of 50 and large numbers of these RNs are expected to retire in the years ahead (independent of the pace and intensity of a jobs recovery)" (AACN, 2010a, p. 4).

9. Nurse educators must rely on

    A. their own "gut feelings" about teaching.

    B. teaching as they were taught by others.

    C. EBT to provide a foundation for novice and experienced faculty.

    D. other healthcare professionals to design education activities/programs to produce a better nursing workforce.

Rationale:

EBT provides a foundation for both novice and experienced faculty to build their knowledge and skills in the nursing education arena on evidence rather than relying on a "gut feeling" or past educational experiences.

10. Competence and expertise are:

    A. needed in the realm of being a nurse educator.

    B. not essential for nursing education.

    C.   a nice approach for nurses at the bedside.

    D.   expected but seldom applied to nursing education.

Rationale:

Just as nurses at the bedside need to be cognizant of new technologies and the need to keep current on EBP, so too does the nurse educator need to maintain competence and expertise in the realm of being a nurse educator.

11.   Barriers to increasing enrollments are

    A.   too many programs from which to choose.

    B.   too many novice faculty who are young in age.

    C.   lack of faculty, clinical sites, and classroom space, as well as budgetary restraints.

    D.   aging of faculty, lack of scholarships, program requirements, and living accommodations.

Rationale:

Barriers to increasing enrollments are lack of faculty, clinical sites, and classroom space, as well as economic budgetary restraints.

12.   Research in nursing education has

    A.   abounded over the years.

    B.   decreased every year.

    C.   little impact on EBT.

    D.   ebbed and flowed in the past.

Rationale:

Research endeavors within nursing education have ebbed and flowed over the last decade. At this time, funding sources and/or streams seem to be opening up for nursing educational research projects.

13.   Evidence-based teaching can be utilized

    A.   only in universities.

    B.   only in community colleges.

    C.   in multiple settings.

    D.   in hospitals only.

Rationale:

Evidence-based teaching has a major impact for nurse educators in clinics, hospitals, schools, home health agencies, and hospice agencies.

Discussion Questions

1. Over the last few semesters, faculty members have investigated the idea of using preceptors for all of the different students. What aspects do the faculty members need to carefully consider in regard to developing an orientation program for the preceptors?

Considerations:

Clinically competent nurses are called upon in many settings to provide the support and practical experience for students to allow for the advancement of the knowledge base. Didactic teaching settings are established to accentuate the cognitive domain of learning. Clinical instructors, preceptors, and coaches are depended upon to translate the cognitive knowledge to the psychomotor and affective domains through application. From the evidence, Modic and Schoessler (2010) identified fours themes that preceptors identified as key areas needing to be strengthened: "(1) learning how to capitalize on teaching moments, (2) applying evidence-based teaching, (3) providing constructive performance feedback, and (4) adapting teaching strategies to match the different learning needs of students" (p. 134). Each of these areas is paramount as orientation programs for preceptors and coaches are established and as preceptors/coaches are supported and developed. Individuals who agree to serve as preceptors and coaches for the next generation of students want to support and develop the novice nurses in a positive and encouraging manner. The idea of "eating our young" is not the feedback that most nurses desire. In reality, the strengthening and championing of the next generation of nurses is the ultimate goal for individuals who accept the responsibility of precepting and coaching student nurses.

2. Nursing faculty members need to consider and experiment with methods of advancing excellence in teaching. Within Valiga's (2010) article, she suggested several ways to accomplish this, such as:

- Constructing open, adaptable curricula that embrace students' learning needs and ignore faculty biases and "sacred cows."
- Engage the learner in ascertaining at least some of the learning objectives for a course or module.
- Embrace the affective domain of learning, rather than ignoring it to concentrate on the cognitive domain of learning only.
- Launch teaching practices based on evidence instead of depending on tradition and/or past experiences.

What other suggestions can you identify that could be used to advance excellence in teaching?

Considerations:

The guest editorial provided by T. Valiga (2010) in the *Journal of Nursing Education* identifies 15 different tactics that could be considered by a faculty member as excellence is sought. Within this editorial, T. Valiga challenges each of us to strive for the next level of nursing education. Each faculty member is encouraged to reach for the stars and break out of the box of traditional nursing education. As the old rules are tested and questioned, new and innovative evidence will be determined that can be used to advance the practice of nursing education to the next level of learning.

Index

1-minute paper, 142, 145